Loving Someone with AuDHD (Autism + ADHD)

The Essential Guide for Partners, Family, and Friends

Mildred Kathryn Hardy

First Edition: 2025

ISBN: 978-1-7643522-0-8

eISBN: 978-1-7643522-1-5

The information in this book is for educational and informational purposes only and is not a substitute for professional medical advice, diagnosis, or treatment. Always seek the advice of your physician, psychiatrist, psychologist, therapist, or other qualified health provider regarding autism spectrum disorder, attention-deficit/hyperactivity disorder, mental health conditions, or relationship concerns.

Every individual and relationship is unique. The strategies and suggestions provided may not be appropriate for all situations, and readers should use their own judgment in applying this information to their specific circumstances. This book provides general relationship guidance and does not replace professional couples therapy, individual counseling, or psychiatric care.

All case examples, scenarios, personal stories, and names presented in this book—including Maya, David, James, Alex, Keisha, Sam, Rebecca, Zoe, Marcus, Aisha, Kelly, Luis, Jenna, Priya, Sara, Leo, Mason, Carmen, Nate, Olivia, Sophie, Emma, Trent, Jordan, Alicia, Jonas, Simone, Tasha, Dev, and all other individuals mentioned—are entirely fictional composites created for illustrative purposes. Any resemblance to actual persons, living or dead, or actual relationships is purely coincidental. These examples are based on common experiences reported in research and clinical settings but do not represent specific individuals.

If you are experiencing relationship crisis, domestic violence, severe mental health symptoms, or thoughts of self-harm, please seek immediate professional help. Contact the National Suicide Prevention Lifeline (988) or the National Domestic Violence Hotline (1-800-799-7233) if you are in crisis.

The publisher and author make no representations or warranties regarding the accuracy or completeness of this book's contents and specifically disclaim any implied warranties of merchantability or fitness for a particular purpose. Neither the publisher nor author shall be liable for any loss of profit or other commercial damages, including special, incidental, consequential, or other damages. All research studies, statistics, and sources cited are provided for informational purposes only. Readers should consult original sources and current research for the most up-to-date information.

The advice and strategies herein may not be suitable for every situation. Readers are encouraged to consult with qualified professionals regarding their specific circumstances. By reading this book, you acknowledge that you understand and agree to this disclaimer.

Table of Contents

Chapter 1: The Paradoxical Brain

You're watching someone you care about make elaborate plans for a weekend getaway, mapping out every detail with precision—only to cancel the entire trip an hour before departure because they suddenly feel overwhelmed. Or maybe they spend three hours passionately explaining their latest interest, then go completely silent for the next three days, avoiding your calls. You're left confused, hurt, and wondering if you did something wrong. The answer is usually no. What you're seeing isn't personal rejection or manipulation. You're witnessing the daily reality of living with AuDHD—a brain caught in an endless tug-of-war between two competing forces.

What AuDHD Actually Means

AuDHD refers to the co-occurrence of autism spectrum disorder and attention-deficit/hyperactivity disorder in the same person. This isn't rare. Research shows that somewhere between 50 and 70 percent of autistic individuals also have ADHD. That's not a small overlap—that's the majority. For years, clinicians didn't even recognize this combination was possible because the diagnostic criteria seemed contradictory. Autism involves preference for routine and predictability. ADHD involves impulsivity and seeking novelty. How could one person have both?

The medical field now understands these conditions aren't opposites—they're two different neurological patterns that can and do coexist. When they do, they create what many AuDHD

1

individuals describe as an internal war. One part of their brain craves structure, order, and predictability. Another part wants spontaneity, novelty, and constant stimulation. These aren't personality quirks. These are neurological differences in how the brain processes information, manages attention, and regulates emotions.

The person you love isn't choosing to be contradictory. They're trying to navigate two competing sets of needs that pull in opposite directions every single day.

The Internal Battle: Structure vs. Spontaneity

Think of the autistic part of the brain as a meticulous project manager. This part wants things organized, scheduled, and predictable. It finds comfort in knowing what comes next. It needs time to prepare for transitions. It wants the same routine because that routine feels safe.

Now think of the ADHD part of the brain as an excitable explorer. This part gets bored easily and needs constant stimulation. It chases interesting ideas down rabbit holes. It says yes to everything because everything sounds exciting in the moment. It struggles to stick with boring but necessary tasks.

These two parts don't work together peacefully. They argue. Constantly. The autistic part says, "We need a plan for Saturday." The ADHD part says, "Plans are boring—let's just see what happens!" The autistic part insists, "We must finish organizing the closet we started." The ADHD part protests, "But that's tedious—look at this new hobby that just caught my attention!"

Your loved one isn't being difficult. They're mediating an exhausting internal negotiation that never ends.

Why Emotional Regulation Is Harder

Here's something you need to know: AuDHD individuals experience more emotional dysregulation than people with autism alone or ADHD alone. The research is clear on this. When you combine the sensory sensitivities and social stress of autism with the impulse control challenges and emotional intensity of ADHD, you get more frequent and more severe meltdowns.

A meltdown isn't a tantrum. It's not manipulation. It's what happens when the nervous system becomes so overwhelmed that the person temporarily loses the ability to regulate their responses. For someone with AuDHD, the threshold for overwhelm is lower because they're already managing two competing sets of challenges.

Small disruptions hit harder. Your loved one might snap at you for moving their coffee mug because the autistic part of their brain needs things in specific places, and the ADHD part already used up all their self-control trying to focus on work that morning. They're not overreacting. They're out of regulatory capacity.

Case Example 1: Maya's Saturday Plans

Maya, 32, loves her partner David. Every Friday evening, she makes detailed plans for Saturday—what time they'll wake up, where they'll get coffee, which museum they'll visit, when they'll have lunch. She prints out directions and double-checks opening hours. David feels touched by her effort and excited about their day together.

Saturday morning arrives. David wakes up ready to go. But Maya is lying in bed, staring at the ceiling, anxiety radiating off her. "I don't think I can do this today," she says quietly. David feels confused and hurt. They had a plan. She made the plan. What changed?

Here's what happened: Maya's autistic brain needed the structure of planning. Making plans felt good. It gave her something to look forward to and reduced uncertainty about the weekend. But overnight, her ADHD brain started feeling trapped by those same plans. The structure that felt comforting on Friday felt suffocating on Saturday. By morning, the thought of following the precise schedule triggered panic rather than excitement.

David didn't understand this for months. He felt jerked around. He thought Maya was being manipulative or didn't actually want to spend time with him. Once Maya explained the internal conflict—how much she genuinely wanted structure and simultaneously felt imprisoned by it—David could see her cancellations differently. Now they build flexibility into plans. They make "maybe" plans with backup options. They check in Saturday morning before committing. The disappointment still happens, but the confusion and hurt have decreased.

Case Example 2: James and the Kitchen Project

James, 28, decided to reorganize the kitchen. He spent two hours creating a detailed plan, labeling shelves, and sorting items by category. His roommate Alex watched this meticulous process with admiration. Finally, James seemed to be tackling the household chaos that usually bothered him.

Three days later, the kitchen was worse than before. Half-empty boxes sat on the counter. Items were scattered everywhere. The new labels were still in their packaging. When Alex asked about it, James looked embarrassed and defensive. "I'll get to it," he muttered. But weeks passed, and the kitchen stayed in disarray.

Alex felt frustrated. If the mess bothered James so much, why couldn't he just finish what he started? This seemed like pure laziness. But here's the reality: the ADHD part of James's brain cannot sustain focus on tedious tasks, even tasks the autistic part of his brain desperately wants completed. The planning stage was interesting and engaging. The actual sorting and labeling became boring after 30 minutes. Once James lost momentum, restarting felt impossible.

James wasn't lazy. He was stuck. His autistic brain couldn't function well in the chaotic kitchen. His ADHD brain couldn't focus long enough to fix it. This is what getting stuck looks like—needing order but lacking the ability to create it through boring, repetitive tasks.

When Alex understood this, they changed their approach. Instead of expecting James to finish the project alone, they worked together in short 15-minute bursts. They made the task more engaging by racing each other and playing music. They accommodated both parts of James's brain—creating the order he needed through a method that maintained his attention.

Case Example 3: Keisha's Communication Pattern

Keisha, 35, has been dating Sam for a year. Sam noticed a pattern but couldn't make sense of it. Some weeks, Keisha texted constantly—long, detailed messages about her day, funny observations, random thoughts. She'd call and talk for hours about philosophy, politics, her childhood memories, Sam's work project. Sam loved these periods. They felt deeply connected.

Then, without warning, Keisha would go quiet. Messages became one-word replies. Phone calls stopped. When they did talk, Keisha seemed distracted and distant. This pattern repeated every few weeks. Sam started to panic during the quiet periods. Had they done something wrong? Was Keisha losing interest? The inconsistency felt destabilizing.

Eventually, Sam asked directly what was happening. Keisha explained that the talkative periods were hyperfocus episodes. When she was interested and engaged, she could talk endlessly. But that level of social output exhausted her autistic brain. After a few days of intense interaction, she needed to retreat and recharge. The silence wasn't rejection—it was recovery.

Sam also learned that Keisha's ADHD made her communication style unpredictable. Sometimes she'd start a text and forget to finish it for hours. Other times, she'd send 15 messages in a row because her brain was moving too fast to organize thoughts into one cohesive message. Understanding this helped Sam stop taking the inconsistency personally.

They developed a system. Keisha would send a short message when she was entering a recharge period: "Brain needs quiet time. Still care about you. Will reconnect when I can." This simple signal helped Sam manage their anxiety and stopped them from spiraling into insecurity during Keisha's silent periods.

The Most Common Paradoxes Decoded

They crave plans but cancel last minute. The planning brings comfort and structure. The execution triggers feelings of constraint and overwhelm. Both needs are real. Both are happening simultaneously.

They're hyperfocused one moment and completely scattered the next. ADHD brains don't regulate attention—they either lock onto something with laser intensity or can't focus at all. There's no middle ground. The autistic need for routine can't override the ADHD attention regulation problems.

They need routine but also novelty. Routines provide safety and reduce decision fatigue. But ADHD brains require stimulation to function. Too much routine leads to understimulation and executive dysfunction. Too much novelty triggers autistic overwhelm.

They talk intensely for hours then go silent for days. Hyperfocus creates periods of intense engagement. But this level of interaction depletes their social and sensory capacity. The silence that follows is necessary recovery, not disinterest.

Reframing: This Is Neurology, Not Character

Here's what you need to accept: these contradictions aren't going away. You can't fix them. You can't love them away or reason them out of existence. The contradictions are built into how your loved one's brain functions.

This doesn't mean your relationship is doomed. It means you need a new framework. Stop expecting consistency. Stop waiting for them to "grow out of" behaviors that confuse you. Stop interpreting contradictions as evidence they don't care about you or the relationship.

Start recognizing these patterns as neurological realities. When your loved one cancels plans they made, they're not being flaky—they're managing an internal conflict you can't see. When they fixate on organizing but can't complete the task, they're not lazy—they're stuck between competing brain demands. When they oscillate between intense connection and withdrawal, they're not playing games—they're managing their limited regulatory capacity.

Your frustration makes sense. Living with unpredictability is hard. But your loved one isn't creating this unpredictability on purpose. They're living with it too, from the inside, with no escape.

The question isn't how to make them more consistent. The question is how to build a relationship structure that accommodates their neurological reality while still meeting your needs. That's what the rest of this book addresses.

Moving Forward

Understanding the internal war doesn't immediately solve the confusion. But it's the necessary first step. You can't accommodate what you don't understand. You can't build helpful systems without recognizing why the contradictions exist.

Your loved one's brain isn't broken. It's wired differently. The ADHD and autism aren't fighting because something is wrong—they're fighting because they're both present and both demanding attention. Your role isn't to pick a side or decide which set of needs is more legitimate. Your role is to recognize that both sets of needs are real and figure out how to support someone managing this exhausting internal negotiation.

The next chapter addresses how this internal conflict affects communication—how your loved one hears what you say, processes what you mean, and expresses what they need. Because if the internal war creates behavioral contradictions, it also creates communication challenges that can make you feel like you're speaking different languages.

Key Takeaways

- AuDHD affects 50-70% of autistic individuals, creating daily conflicts between the need for structure (autism) and spontaneity (ADHD)

- The contradictions you observe aren't personality flaws or manipulation—they're neurological realities of managing two competing sets of brain demands

- AuDHD individuals experience more severe emotional dysregulation and meltdowns than those with autism or ADHD alone

- Common paradoxes include craving plans but canceling them, needing both routine and novelty, and alternating between intense connection and withdrawal

- The "getting stuck" phenomenon happens when the autistic brain needs order but the ADHD brain can't sustain attention on boring organizational tasks

- Your loved one lives with this internal conflict constantly—they're not creating unpredictability to frustrate you

- Building accommodations requires understanding these neurological patterns, not trying to eliminate or "fix" them

Chapter 2: The Hidden Language

Translating What They Say, What They Mean, and What They Can't Express

Communication breakdowns don't happen because your AuDHD loved one doesn't care about you. They happen because you're essentially speaking related but distinct languages. You both use the same words, but those words carry different meanings in your respective brains. You both send and receive messages, but the encoding and decoding processes work differently. This creates a communication gap that feels frustrating for both of you—you feel unheard and misunderstood, and so do they.

The Double Frustration Problem

Research on neurodiverse relationships shows a consistent pattern. Neurotypical partners report feeling like their neurodivergent partner doesn't care enough or isn't trying hard enough. Meanwhile, neurodivergent partners report feeling like their neurotypical partner lacks patience and is impossible to please. Both partners feel misunderstood. Both are often correct in their perception that the other doesn't fully understand them.

This isn't about who's right or wrong. It's about recognizing that you process communication through different neurological filters. What seems obvious to you isn't obvious to them. What feels like clear communication to them might feel confusing or inadequate to you. Neither perspective is more valid. They're just different.

The solution isn't for one person to entirely adopt the other's communication style. The solution is developing a shared communication system that accounts for both styles.

The Literal Thinking Challenge

Autistic individuals process language more literally than neurotypical people. This isn't a cute quirk or something they can turn off when it's inconvenient. It's how their brains process language.

If you say, "I'm starving," a neurotypical person understands you're hungry, not actually dying from starvation. An autistic person might take this literally and feel confused about why you're being dramatic about missing one meal. If you say, "Can you take out the trash?" a neurotypical person hears this as a request. An autistic person might respond "Yes" and then not take out the trash—because you asked if they *can* do it, not if they *will* do it.

Idioms and sarcasm create particular confusion. "It's raining cats and dogs" doesn't actually involve animals falling from the sky. "Oh great, that's just what I needed" said sarcastically means the opposite of its literal meaning. But autistic brains process the literal words first. They have to consciously translate figurative language, and that translation doesn't always happen successfully, especially under stress.

This matters in relationships because indirect communication creates constant miscommunication. If you're upset and say, "I'm fine," expecting your partner to recognize your tone indicates you're not actually fine, you're setting up frustration. Your autistic partner might take "I'm fine" at face value and move on, leaving you feeling ignored when they genuinely didn't receive the message you thought you sent.

ADHD Communication Patterns

The ADHD part of your loved one's brain creates different communication challenges. ADHD affects working memory, attention regulation, and impulse control—all of which directly impact communication.

Your partner might interrupt you mid-sentence. This isn't rudeness. Their brain had a thought in response to what you said, and the ADHD impulse control deficit means the thought came out of their mouth before they consciously decided to speak. By the time they finish their thought, they've forgotten what you were saying.

They might seem distracted during important conversations. They're not trying to dismiss what you're saying. Their ADHD brain struggles to maintain focus on things that aren't immediately stimulating, even things they care deeply about. Sitting still and tracking a long conversation requires sustained attention their brain struggles to provide.

They might forget conversations entirely. Not because those conversations didn't matter, but because ADHD affects memory consolidation. Information has to make it from short-term to long-term memory. For ADHD brains, this process is less reliable. They might genuinely have no memory of a conversation you remember clearly.

They might start conversations and then abandon them. You're talking about dinner plans, and suddenly they're telling you about something they saw on social media. The ADHD brain made an associative leap—something you said connected to another thought, which connected to another, and now they're three topics away from where you started.

What Works: Direct and Explicit Communication

The most effective communication strategy with AuDHD individuals is radical directness. This feels awkward to many neurotypical people. You've been socialized to soften requests, hint at needs, and avoid being "too direct." That socialization works against you here.

Instead of: "Do you think maybe at some point you could possibly help with the dishes?"

Try: "Please wash the dishes tonight after dinner."

Instead of: "I've noticed the trash is getting pretty full..."

Try: "I need you to take out the trash now."

Instead of: "Are you okay? You seem quiet."

Try: "You've been quieter than usual. I'm worried something is wrong. Can you tell me if you're okay or if you need space?"

Direct communication isn't rude. It's clear. It eliminates the guesswork and subtext that neurotypical brains process automatically but neurodivergent brains often miss.

Case Example 1: The Birthday Surprise Disaster

Rachel wanted to do something special for her partner Morgan's birthday. She'd been dropping hints for weeks: mentioning how much she loved surprise parties, showing Morgan photos of friend's birthday celebrations, asking seemingly casual questions about Morgan's schedule for their birthday weekend. Rachel felt she was clearly communicating her expectations.

Morgan's birthday arrived. Rachel had secretly organized a surprise party. She'd invited Morgan's friends, decorated their apartment, and arranged for Morgan's favorite food. When Morgan came home, everyone jumped out yelling "Surprise!"

Morgan's face went white. They turned around and walked out of the apartment without a word.

Rachel was devastated. She'd worked so hard. Morgan came back an hour later, overwhelmed and apologetic. They explained that they had no idea Rachel wanted a party. The hints Rachel dropped didn't register as hints—they seemed like random comments about other people's experiences. Morgan hates surprises because their autistic brain needs time to prepare for social situations. Being ambushed by unexpected guests and noise triggered an immediate shutdown response.

Rachel felt awful. Morgan felt guilty. But both learned something critical: hinting doesn't work. Now when Rachel wants to plan something, she asks directly. "Your birthday is coming up. I'd like to do something special. What would feel good to you?" Morgan can then communicate their needs clearly without Rachel having to guess.

Case Example 2: The "Just Checking In" Text

Devon sent their partner Alex a text: "Hey, just checking in. How's your day going?" This felt like a caring, low-pressure message to Devon. Alex didn't respond for six hours. When they finally replied, it was one word: "Fine."

Devon felt hurt. Alex clearly didn't want to talk to them. Why even be in a relationship if Alex couldn't be bothered to have a simple conversation?

Here's what actually happened: Alex was in a period of ADHD hyperfocus at work. They saw the text notification but thought, "I'll respond after I finish this task." Then they forgot the text existed. Six hours later, they remembered and felt panicked. They'd neglected their partner! They needed to respond immediately! But they couldn't remember what the text said or what Devon wanted to know. They opened it, saw "How's your day going?" and their ADHD brain went blank. How do you summarize six hours? They were overwhelmed, so they sent "Fine" because at least that was a response.

When Devon explained they felt ignored, Alex was surprised. They weren't ignoring Devon—they were struggling with working memory and response paralysis. Devon learned to send more specific texts: "I miss you and want to hear about your day when you have time. No rush to respond." Alex learned to set phone reminders to check messages. They also explained to Devon that short responses didn't mean disinterest—sometimes they just meant "I saw this and don't have processing capacity for more right now."

Case Example 3: The Shutdown vs. Silent Treatment Confusion

After an argument, Tomás noticed his partner Jordan went completely silent. Not just quiet—silent. Jordan stopped responding to questions, stopped making eye contact, and retreated to another room. Tomás interpreted this as the silent treatment, a manipulative punishment he'd experienced in past relationships. His frustration grew. They couldn't resolve anything if Jordan refused to communicate.

But Jordan wasn't giving Tomás the silent treatment. Jordan was experiencing a shutdown. Shutdowns happen when an autistic person's nervous system becomes so overwhelmed that they temporarily lose the ability to process or produce language. It's not a choice. It's a neurological response to stress.

During arguments, Jordan's brain became overloaded with emotional information, social demands, and the need to formulate responses quickly. The system overloaded and shut down. In that state, Jordan physically couldn't speak or process spoken language effectively. Trying to continue the argument would only extend the shutdown.

Once Tomás understood the difference between a shutdown and deliberate silence, he could respond appropriately. Now when Jordan goes silent during conflict, Tomás recognizes it as a sign they need a break. He says, "I can see you're overwhelmed. I'm going to step away for a while. We'll come back to this when you're ready." This removes the pressure and gives Jordan's nervous system time to regulate. Later, when Jordan has recovered, they finish the conversation more productively.

Reading Social Cues and Tone

Neurotypical communication relies heavily on nonverbal information. Your tone of voice, facial expression, and body language carry as much meaning as your words—sometimes more. You can say "I'm fine" in a tone that clearly means you're not fine. A neurotypical person picks up that contradiction automatically.

Autistic brains don't process these nonverbal cues as efficiently. Your partner might miss your irritated expression entirely. They might hear your sarcastic tone but not understand that the sarcasm reverses the literal meaning of your words. They might not notice you're upset until you explicitly say, "I'm upset."

This creates situations where you feel obvious in your emotional state, and they seem oblivious. You're radiating anger, and they're asking what you want for dinner. You're clearly hurt, and they're chatting about something unrelated. They're not emotionally insensitive. They're not seeing the nonverbal cues you're broadcasting.

The solution is naming your emotions explicitly. "I'm feeling frustrated right now because the dishes are still in the sink." "I'm hurt that you forgot our plans." "I'm angry and need some time before we discuss this." This feels awkward and unnaturally direct. But it works. It gives your partner the information their brain isn't automatically extracting from your facial expressions and tone.

Practical Scripts for Difficult Conversations

Difficult conversations require extra structure. Here are templates that account for AuDHD communication needs:

For bringing up a problem:

"I need to talk about [specific issue]. Is now a good time, or should we schedule a time later today/tomorrow?" This gives them time to prepare mentally rather than being ambushed.

"I feel [specific emotion] when [specific behavior] happens. I need [specific change]. Can we talk about how to make that happen?" This provides clear information about the problem and desired solution.

For expressing needs:

"I need [specific thing] by [specific time]. Can you do that?" This creates clarity and allows them to say yes or no rather than agreeing to something vague they might forget.

For checking understanding:

"Can you tell me what you heard me say? I want to make sure I communicated clearly." This catches miscommunication before it creates bigger problems.

For managing conflict:

"I'm getting overwhelmed and need a break. Can we pause this conversation for [specific amount of time] and come back to it?" This prevents shutdowns and meltdowns by allowing regulation breaks.

The Power of Scheduled Conversations

One of the most effective strategies is scheduling important conversations. This sounds unromantic. Shouldn't you be able to talk about important things when they come up? In theory, yes. In practice, ambushing your AuDHD partner with serious conversations often goes poorly.

Their brain needs preparation time. Springing a serious discussion on them triggers anxiety and makes it harder for them to process and respond effectively. Scheduling a conversation allows their brain to prepare. They can think through what they want to say. They can mentally rehearse the interaction. They can ensure they're in a good headspace for a difficult discussion.

"Can we talk about our vacation plans this Saturday morning after breakfast?" works better than starting a conversation about vacation plans while they're hyperfocused on work. "I'd like to schedule time this weekend to discuss our finances. What time works for you?" works better than bringing up money concerns randomly.

This takes some of the spontaneity out of communication. But it dramatically improves the quality of the conversations you do have.

What Silence Really Means

Not all silence means the same thing. Your AuDHD loved one might be silent because they're:

- Experiencing a shutdown and can't process language

- Hyperfocused on something and not registering you're speaking

- Overwhelmed and needing sensory quiet

- Processing what you said and formulating a response (this takes longer for them)

- Struggling to find words to express complex feelings

- Needing space to regulate their emotions

They might also be silent because they're upset with you. But that's just one option among many. Before assuming silence means anger or disinterest, check. "I notice you're quiet. Are you okay, or do you need space?" A direct question gets you a clearer answer than guessing.

Building Your Shared Language

Every relationship requires developing shared communication patterns. For neurodiverse relationships, this process needs to be more conscious and explicit. You're not just learning each other's preferences—you're building a bridge between different neurological processing styles.

This means having conversations about how you communicate. What does your partner need from you when they're overwhelmed? How should you indicate you're upset? What's the best way to bring up problems? How can you tell the difference between them needing space and them withdrawing?

These conversations feel awkward at first. You're making explicit what usually stays implicit. But this explicit shared language becomes the foundation for effective communication. You develop your own system that accounts for both your needs.

Looking Ahead

Understanding communication differences reduces frustration, but you still need to manage the social energy dynamics that affect how much communication your partner can handle. The next chapter addresses why your partner oscillates between intense connection and withdrawal—and how to maintain closeness without burning them out.

Key Takeaways

- Communication breakdowns happen because neurotypical and neurodivergent brains process language differently, not because either partner doesn't care

- Autistic brains process language literally—idioms, sarcasm, and indirect communication create confusion rather than clarity

- ADHD affects working memory, attention, and impulse control, leading to forgotten conversations, interruptions, and seeming distraction

- Direct, explicit communication works best—replace hints and subtext with clear statements of needs and feelings

- Shutdowns are neurological responses to overwhelm, not deliberate silent treatment or manipulation

- Autistic individuals often miss nonverbal cues like facial expressions and tone, so naming emotions explicitly prevents misunderstanding

- Scheduling important conversations rather than "springing" them allows preparation time and improves discussion quality

- Building a shared communication system requires explicit conversations about what each person needs to communicate effectively

Chapter 3: The Social Energy Roller Coaster

Understanding the Push-Pull of Connection and Withdrawal

Your partner spent last weekend attached to you—talking for hours, making plans, wanting physical closeness, actively engaged in every activity. You felt connected and happy. This week, they've barely responded to your texts. When you're together, they seem distant and distracted. You try to initiate conversation, and they give one-word answers. You suggest activities, and they decline. What changed? Did you do something wrong? Are they losing interest?

Probably not. What you're experiencing is the AuDHD social energy cycle. Your partner isn't playing games or sending mixed signals. They're managing limited social and sensory capacity that fluctuates in ways you can't see from the outside.

The Exhaustion of Masking

Most autistic individuals learn to mask—they suppress their natural autistic behaviors and mimic neurotypical social behavior. They make eye contact even though it's uncomfortable. They follow conversation scripts they've memorized. They monitor their volume and tone. They force themselves to smile and nod at appropriate times. They pretend to care about small talk. They hide their stims. They act interested in topics that bore them.

Masking isn't a conscious choice most of the time. It's a survival strategy learned through years of negative feedback for being "too weird" or "too different." Your partner likely started masking in childhood and now does it automatically around most people.

But masking is exhausting. Spending time with neurotypical people who expect neurotypical behavior requires constant conscious effort. Every social interaction drains their capacity. They're not just participating in conversation—they're simultaneously monitoring their behavior, adjusting their responses, and suppressing their natural reactions.

Time with close partners sometimes allows them to unmask. They can be themselves without constantly self-monitoring. But even in close relationships, social interaction requires energy. And if they're masking in other contexts (work, family events, running errands), they come home with an empty capacity tank.

When you see your partner withdraw, they're not rejecting you. They're out of social energy. They need time alone to recover their capacity before they can engage again.

The ADHD Hyperfocus Phase

Early in relationships, AuDHD individuals often seem intensely present and connected. This isn't fake. It's ADHD hyperfocus. When something or someone is new and interesting, the ADHD brain locks in. Your partner can spend hours talking, texting, planning, engaging. They think about you constantly. They want to be with you all the time. This phase feels exciting for both partners.

But hyperfocus doesn't last. Eventually, the relationship becomes familiar rather than novel. The ADHD brain requires novelty to maintain that level of engagement. When the hyperfocus phase ends, your partner's attention naturally redistributes to other things. They still care about you. They still value the relationship. But they can't maintain the same intensity of focus they had initially.

This shift often happens around the same time the relationship gets more serious. Your partner seems less engaged right when you're getting more attached. This timing makes the change feel personal. You interpret their reduced intensity as reduced interest. But they're not pulling away—their ADHD brain is returning to its normal attention regulation pattern after an unsustainable hyperfocus period.

Understanding this pattern helps you not take the shift personally. The early intensity wasn't the "real" relationship—it was the unsustainable hyperfocus version. The steadier, less intense connection that follows is actually more sustainable long-term.

Case Example 1: The Weekend Whiplash

Sofia and her girlfriend Lauren had been dating for eight months. Every few weeks, they'd have an incredible weekend together. They'd stay up late talking about everything, make love, cook together, take long walks, share their dreams and fears. Sofia felt deeply connected during these weekends. This was the relationship she wanted.

Then Monday would arrive, and Lauren would essentially disappear. She'd text Sofia once a day with minimal content. She'd decline invitations to get together. When Sofia would express feeling ignored, Lauren would seem confused and distant. This pattern repeated every few weeks, and Sofia couldn't understand it.

Finally, Sofia asked directly what was happening. Lauren explained that the intense weekends completely depleted her. After two days of sustained social interaction, even with someone she loved, her autistic brain needed recovery time. The masking required—even though she felt safe with Sofia, she still monitored her behavior more than when she was alone—

exhausted her. She needed several days of minimal interaction to recharge before she could engage fully again.

Sofia initially felt hurt. Didn't Lauren want to spend time with her? Lauren did. But she also needed alone time to function. They negotiated a new pattern. Instead of occasional intense weekends followed by days of distance, they scheduled shorter but more frequent time together. Lauren could manage three-hour periods of connection without depleting herself entirely. They also established a signal: when Lauren texted "low battery," Sofia understood she was entering a recharge period and wouldn't take the reduced contact personally.

This change didn't eliminate all frustration. Sofia still sometimes wanted more time than Lauren could give. But understanding the pattern helped Sofia stop interpreting Lauren's withdrawal as rejection. The withdrawal was recovery, not disinterest.

Case Example 2: The Party Circuit Crash

Marcus loved his boyfriend Isaac's enthusiasm for social activities. In the first six months they dated, Isaac eagerly attended every party, dinner, and event Marcus suggested. Isaac seemed to genuinely enjoy meeting Marcus's friends, going to social gatherings, being part of Marcus's active social life.

Then Isaac started declining invitations. First occasionally, then frequently. Within a few months, Isaac rarely wanted to attend social events. When he did come, he'd often leave early or spend the evening looking uncomfortable. Marcus felt disappointed and confused. Had Isaac been faking interest in his friends?

No. Isaac had been hyperfocusing. The new relationship was exciting, and his ADHD brain was all in. Meeting Marcus's friends felt interesting. Going to parties provided novelty. He genuinely enjoyed these activities initially.

But several factors shifted. First, the novelty wore off. Once Isaac had met Marcus's friend group, subsequent gatherings became repetitive rather than stimulating. His ADHD brain started finding these events boring. Second, the sustained social schedule accumulated exhaustion. Isaac's autistic brain was masking heavily at every event, and the social battery never fully recharged between gatherings.

When Isaac tried to explain this, Marcus felt rejected. If Isaac loved him, wouldn't he want to be part of his social life? Marcus interpreted Isaac's reduced participation as pulling away from the relationship. But Isaac wasn't pulling away from Marcus—he was protecting his limited social capacity.

They found a compromise. Isaac attended the events most important to Marcus but skipped others without guilt. At parties, they established a signal for when Isaac needed to leave, and Marcus would either leave with him or stay while Isaac went home. Marcus also started scheduling one-on-one time with Isaac that didn't involve group social settings. This gave them connection time that didn't deplete Isaac's social energy as rapidly.

Case Example 3: The Text Message Mystery

Yuki sent their partner Chris detailed, thoughtful texts every day. They shared articles, memes, observations about their day, questions about Chris's interests. The texts were engaging and showed genuine interest in Chris's life.

Then Yuki would suddenly go days without texting. Chris would send messages and get no response. When Chris asked if everything was okay, Yuki would send brief reassurances but no explanation. After a few days, Yuki would return to the detailed texting pattern. Chris felt confused and anxious. Was Yuki upset? Losing interest? Playing some kind of game?

When they finally discussed it, Yuki explained the pattern. During talkative periods, Yuki was hyperfocusing on the relationship. Their ADHD brain was engaged, and texting came easily. During quiet periods, Yuki wasn't upset or distant—they were either hyperfocusing on something else (work projects, hobbies, family matters) and genuinely forgetting to check their phone, or they were in a period of social exhaustion where even texting felt like too much interaction.

The silence wasn't intentional communication. It was the natural result of ADHD attention shifting and autistic social capacity fluctuating. Yuki still cared about Chris during the quiet periods. They just didn't have the capacity to maintain constant communication.

Chris struggled with this. They needed more consistent communication to feel secure in the relationship. They negotiated a minimum: even during low-energy periods, Yuki would send one brief check-in text daily. This didn't require long messages or deep conversation. Just "Thinking of you, low energy today" or "Busy with work, love you." These brief messages helped Chris feel connected without requiring Yuki to maintain the unsustainable intense communication pattern.

Recognizing the Warning Signs

Learning to recognize when your partner is approaching social capacity limits helps prevent total withdrawals. Watch for:

- Shorter responses to questions
- Less initiation of conversation or activities
- More time alone or in quiet activities
- Increased irritability or sensitivity
- More frequent stims or self-soothing behaviors

- Declining invitations they previously would have accepted

- Physical indicators like tension, fatigue, or headaches

These signs mean their capacity is getting low. Pushing for more interaction at this point often triggers complete shutdown or meltdown. Recognizing early signs allows you to suggest a break before they hit empty.

Creating Sustainable Social Routines

Sustainable social routines account for both partners' needs. Your AuDHD partner needs some social interaction—they care about you and want connection. But they need that interaction structured in ways that don't constantly deplete them.

What works varies by person, but common patterns include:

- Regular, predictable together time rather than sporadic intense periods

- Scheduled alone time that's protected and guilt-free

- Shorter, more frequent interactions rather than marathon sessions

- Low-demand connection options (watching TV together, parallel activities) that provide presence without requiring active engagement

- Clear communication about capacity levels

You might schedule three evenings together per week rather than expecting daily connection. You might have a weekly date night but also weekly solo nights. You might develop activities you can do in the same space without constant interaction—you read while they work on a hobby, sharing space without demanding conversation.

These structures feel less spontaneous than stereotypical romantic relationships. But they're more sustainable. Your partner can anticipate social demands and manage their energy accordingly.

The Compromise Day Strategy

Some couples use "compromise days" to balance planning needs with spontaneity needs. One week, Partner A plans the day completely. Partner B agrees to go along with the plan without requiring flexibility. The next week, Partner B leads, and Partner A follows.

This accommodates both the autistic need for predictability and the ADHD need for spontaneity. The planning partner gets structure. The following partner gets to not think about decisions. You alternate who gets which need met.

During this time, you might also build in structured spontaneity—planning the framework but leaving details flexible. "Saturday afternoon we'll do an activity together, location and timing to be decided Saturday morning based on how we feel." This provides structure (we have plans) and flexibility (we'll decide details later).

Staying Connected During Recharge Periods

Your partner needs alone time, but you need connection. How do you maintain closeness when they're withdrawn?

First, reframe what connection means. Connection doesn't always require active engagement. Your partner reading in the same room while you watch TV is connection. A brief text saying "thinking of you" is connection. Them doing their hobby while you do yours in shared space is connection.

Second, develop low-demand connection rituals. A quick hug before bed. A goodnight text. Sharing one highlight from your day. These small touches maintain connection without requiring the energy of deep conversation or active engagement.

Third, respect the recharge period. Don't pressure them to engage before they're ready. Trying to force interaction when they don't have capacity creates resentment and extends the recharge period. Giving them space actually helps them recover faster and return to connection sooner.

Managing Your Own Needs

You have legitimate needs for connection and attention. Your partner's limited capacity doesn't erase your needs. The question is how to meet your needs without depleting your partner.

You might need to get some social and emotional needs met outside the relationship. Close friendships, family relationships, therapy, support groups—these can provide connection and attention when your partner is in a recharge period.

You might need to advocate for minimum connection thresholds. "I understand you need alone time, but I need at least one check-in text per day to feel secure." "I understand you're socially exhausted, but I need at least one date night per week." These minimum thresholds give you what you need without requiring your partner to maintain unsustainable intensity.

You might need to adjust your expectations. If you're someone who thrives on constant communication and togetherness, you might not be compatible with someone whose capacity is more limited. That's okay. Understanding incompatibility early is better than years of frustration trying to change fundamental patterns.

The Balance Point

The goal isn't making your partner more consistently available or making yourself need less connection. The goal is finding a balance point that mostly meets both your needs most of the time.

This balance will always involve compromise. Your partner might engage more than feels comfortable sometimes. You might accept less connection than you prefer sometimes. Perfect accommodation of both partners' needs all the time isn't realistic. But you can build a relationship structure where both partners feel mostly satisfied and no one is constantly depleted or resentful.

This requires ongoing communication. Capacity fluctuates. What worked last month might not work this month. Regular check-ins about what's working and what needs adjustment keep the relationship functional as circumstances change.

Bridging Forward

Understanding social energy dynamics helps make sense of the push-pull pattern, but it doesn't address the practical challenges of daily life management. The next chapter examines executive function differences—how time blindness, task initiation struggles, and organizational challenges show up in relationships, and how to support these areas without becoming your partner's manager.

Key Takeaways

- Social interaction requires masking and depletes energy faster for AuDHD individuals, even in close relationships

- The early relationship hyperfocus phase creates unsustainable intensity that naturally decreases as novelty wears off

- Withdrawal and reduced communication usually signal low social capacity, not reduced interest or rejection

- Warning signs of depleted capacity include shorter responses, increased irritability, and declining invitations

- Sustainable routines involve regular, predictable connection time with protected alone time for recharging

- Low-demand connection options (parallel activities, brief check-ins) maintain closeness without depleting capacity

- Meeting some social needs outside the relationship prevents partner burnout and allows them to recharge

- Finding a balance point requires ongoing communication and compromise from both partners

Chapter 4: Time, Tasks, and the Invisible Clock

Supporting Executive Function Without Becoming the Manager

The dishes have been sitting in the sink for three days. Your partner walked past them twenty times. They mentioned how much the mess bothers them. They even said they'd handle it "later today." But later never comes. You're standing in the kitchen again, staring at those same dishes, feeling a familiar frustration building. You could just wash them yourself—it would take five minutes. But you've already done this dance too many times. You wash the dishes, fold the laundry, pay the bills, schedule the appointments, and somehow you've become the household manager while your partner plays the role of forgetful teenager. This wasn't what you signed up for. And yet, here you are, wondering if you should just do it yourself or wait and see if they actually follow through this time.

This scenario plays out in thousands of homes every day. The neurotypical partner gradually absorbs more and more responsibility. The AuDHD partner seems unable to manage basic adulting tasks. Resentment builds on both sides. You feel like you're parenting your partner. They feel inadequate and criticized. Neither of you wants this dynamic, but you keep sliding into it anyway.

The problem isn't laziness. The problem is executive function deficits combined with something called time blindness. Understanding these neurological challenges doesn't make the dishes magically clean themselves. But it does help you build systems that work instead of constantly battling against your partner's brain.

What Time Blindness Actually Looks Like

Time blindness means your partner's internal clock doesn't work the way yours does. You can look at a task and estimate how long it takes. You know that showering takes about 15 minutes, grocery shopping takes an hour, and driving across town requires 30 minutes. Your brain tracks time passing and alerts you when you need to transition to the next activity.

Your partner's brain doesn't do this automatically. They start a task and genuinely lose track of time. Three hours vanish in what feels like 30 minutes. Or they overestimate how long something takes—they think a simple errand requires the entire afternoon when it actually needs 20 minutes. Their brain can't accurately perceive time passing or estimate task duration.

This creates chronic lateness. They're not disrespecting you when they're late. They genuinely thought they had more time. They started getting ready "in plenty of time" but didn't account for how long each step actually takes. They got distracted during the process and lost 15 minutes without realizing it. By the time they check the clock, they're already late.

It also creates the "waiting mode" problem. If your partner has an appointment at 2 PM, their brain might refuse to start any task before then. They can't relax or be productive. They just wait, watching the clock, afraid to start anything because "we have to leave soon." Even if the appointment is four hours away.

Time blindness affects task completion too. Your partner starts organizing the closet, thinking it'll take an hour. Four hours later, they're still sorting clothes, exhausted and nowhere near finished. They had no way to accurately gauge the task scope.

Now they're stuck—too tired to continue, too bothered by the mess to leave it undone.

You can't see time blindness from the outside. You just see someone who's always late, who can't finish projects, who seems to waste time and then panic about being behind. But they're not choosing this. Their brain literally cannot track and estimate time the way yours does.

Executive Function: The Brain's Management System

Executive function refers to the mental processes that help you plan, organize, prioritize, start tasks, stay focused, remember steps, shift between activities, and manage time. It's your brain's management system. And in AuDHD individuals, this system has significant glitches.

Breaking down complex tasks into steps—executive function handles that. Your brain automatically thinks "clean the kitchen" and creates a plan: clear the counters, load the dishwasher, wipe surfaces, sweep the floor. Your partner's brain doesn't automatically create that plan. They see "clean the kitchen" as one overwhelming blob of work. They don't know where to start, so they don't start at all.

Prioritizing tasks—executive function does this. You look at your to-do list and intuitively know what needs to happen first. Your partner looks at the same list and feels paralyzed because everything seems equally urgent and equally impossible. They can't rank the tasks, so they either do nothing or hyperfocus on the least important item because it's the only one their brain can grab onto.

Initiating tasks—this requires executive function. You decide to do something and then you do it. Your partner decides to do something and then... nothing happens. They're stuck. They know they need to start. They want to start. But the signal from "decision" to "action" doesn't fire. They're frozen not by lack of motivation but by a neurological inability to initiate the task.

Switching between tasks—executive function manages this too. You finish one activity and smoothly transition to the next. Your partner finishes one activity and either gets stuck hyperfocusing on the next one or can't figure out what to do next at all. The transition points become obstacles.

Working memory—executive function maintains this. You can hold multiple pieces of information in your head simultaneously. Your partner struggles with this. You tell them three things you need from the store. By the time they arrive at the store, they remember one item and vaguely feel like there were others but can't recall what they were.

None of this is laziness. These are neurological differences in how the brain manages cognitive tasks. Your partner isn't choosing to be disorganized or forgetful. Their brain's management system legitimately doesn't function the way yours does.

Case Example 1: The Bill Payment Disaster

Marcus and his wife Diane had been married for five years. Diane had ADHD and autism, and Marcus had gradually taken over all the household management. He paid bills, scheduled appointments, maintained the calendar, organized their finances. He told himself he was helping. But he was also exhausted and resentful.

One month, Marcus decided to test Diane. He didn't pay the electric bill. He wanted to see if she'd notice, if she'd take responsibility, if she'd step up. She didn't. The electricity got shut off. Diane was shocked and embarrassed. Marcus was furious. How could she not notice? How could she be so irresponsible?

Here's what Diane experienced: She had no system for tracking bills. She didn't know when they were due or how much they cost. Marcus had always handled it, so she never learned the process. She had vague awareness that bills existed, but her brain couldn't hold that information as an active priority. Out of sight meant out of mind. The executive function required to monitor due dates, remember to check accounts, and initiate payment simply wasn't happening.

Marcus thought he was teaching Diane a lesson about responsibility. Actually, he set her up to fail. He withdrew support without creating a system she could use. He expected her to suddenly develop executive function skills she didn't have.

They needed a different approach. They set up automatic bill payments so Diane didn't need to remember due dates. They created a shared calendar with notifications. They built systems that compensated for Diane's executive function challenges rather than expecting her brain to suddenly work differently. Marcus still monitored the systems, but Diane wasn't completely dependent. And Marcus wasn't drowning in tasks that could be automated.

The key wasn't Marcus doing everything or Diane magically becoming organized. The key was building external structures that worked with Diane's brain instead of against it.

Case Example 2: The Unfinished Projects Everywhere

Aisha loved her boyfriend Jamal, but his unfinished projects drove her to distraction. The bathroom renovation sat half-complete for six months. The garage organization system consisted of labeled boxes that were never actually filled. The meal prep plan lasted two weeks before falling apart.

Jamal would get excited about a project, plan it meticulously, start enthusiastically—and then abandon it partway through.

Aisha felt like she was living in a house full of half-realized intentions. She tried encouraging him. She tried helping. She tried ignoring it. Nothing worked.

Jamal felt ashamed. He knew the projects bothered Aisha. He wanted to finish them. But once the interesting planning phase ended, his ADHD brain couldn't maintain focus on the boring execution phase. And his autistic brain, which desperately wanted the completed organization, couldn't override the ADHD attention regulation problems.

The bathroom renovation stalled because tiling was repetitive and tedious. His brain could not sustain attention on it. Every time he thought about finishing, he felt overwhelmed by how boring it would be. So he avoided it entirely.

The garage organization failed because filling boxes wasn't stimulating enough. The meal prep fell apart because cooking the same things every week became monotonous. In every case, the initial planning sparked interest, but the follow-through required sustained attention on tasks his brain found unstimulating.

Aisha and Jamal found a solution: breaking projects into very small chunks and building in external accountability. Instead of "tile the bathroom," they made it "tile one square foot per day." Jamal could manage 15 minutes of tiling. He couldn't manage four hours. They also hired help for the most boring parts— someone else finished the bathroom tiling, and Jamal completed the trim work, which he found interesting.

For ongoing tasks like meal prep, they simplified. Instead of elaborate plans Jamal couldn't maintain, they created a rotation of five easy meals and accepted that was good enough. They let go of the garage organization fantasy and put everything in large unlabeled bins. Good enough became acceptable. Aisha had to adjust her standards, and Jamal had to accept his limitations.

Case Example 3: The Calendar Catastrophe

Chen and his partner Riley had constant conflicts about scheduling. Riley would agree to plans and then forget completely. Chen would remind Riley about appointments, only to discover Riley double-booked. Riley would promise to remember important dates and then be blindsided when they arrived.

Chen felt disrespected. If Riley cared, wouldn't they remember? Riley felt overwhelmed and inadequate. They didn't want to forget. Their brain just wouldn't hold the information.

The problem was working memory. Riley's ADHD brain struggled to maintain information over time. They'd genuinely intend to remember an appointment. Five minutes later, it vanished from their awareness. They'd agree to plans and then have no memory of the conversation. They'd write things down and then forget where they wrote them.

Chen was using a paper calendar. Riley needed digital systems with multiple reminders. They switched to a shared Google Calendar with notifications. Riley got alerts one week before, one day before, and one hour before any event. This outsourced the remembering to technology instead of relying on Riley's faulty working memory.

They also implemented a new rule: no verbal agreements. Any plan had to go directly into the calendar immediately or it didn't exist. This felt rigid to Chen at first. But it eliminated the pattern of Riley agreeing to things and then forgetting. If Riley couldn't add it to the calendar right then, they'd say "I need to check my calendar before I agree," which was honest and functional.

Riley also started blocking out transition time. If they had a 2 PM appointment, they blocked out 1:30 to 2 PM for preparation and travel. This compensated for time blindness and reduced chronic lateness. The systems didn't fix Riley's executive function deficits, but they worked around them.

The Parent Trap and How It Destroys Relationships

Here's what happens in many neurodiverse relationships: the neurotypical partner gradually takes on more responsibility. They handle tasks their AuDHD partner struggles with. This seems helpful initially. But over time, the dynamic becomes toxic.

You start treating your partner like a child who needs supervision. You remind them of tasks. You check if they've completed things. You organize their life. You speak to them in a tone you'd use with a forgetful teenager. You express disappointment when they fail to meet expectations. You feel like you're carrying the entire household.

Your partner starts feeling incompetent and criticized. They hear your reminders as nagging. They feel your disappointment as judgment. They become defensive and resentful. They stop trying because they assume you'll just take over anyway. Or they avoid tasks entirely to escape the shame of failing at them.

Both partners end up miserable. You're exhausted from managing everything. They're demoralized from feeling inadequate. You've created learned helplessness—your partner becomes less capable because you've made them dependent on you.

This happens with good intentions. You see your partner struggling. You want to help. You step in. But stepping in too much removes the opportunity for your partner to develop compensatory strategies. And it positions you as the parent managing an incompetent child rather than partners managing a household together.

Breaking out of this pattern requires conscious effort. You need to stop doing things for your partner that they can do themselves, even if they do them differently or imperfectly. You need to let them experience consequences sometimes. You need to resist the urge to take over when they're struggling. And you need to change how you communicate—from nagging and criticizing to collaborating and problem-solving.

Spotting Codependency Before It Takes Over

Codependency in neurodiverse relationships often looks like devotion. You're not trying to control your partner. You're trying to help. But if you look closely, you might notice warning signs that your help has crossed into unhealthy territory.

You feel responsible for your partner's failures. When they forget an appointment, you feel like you should have reminded them. When they don't complete a task, you feel obligated to finish it. You've taken ownership of their executive function challenges.

You're doing things they could do themselves. You call to schedule their doctor appointments because "they never get around to it." You manage all the finances because "they're bad with money." You organize their workspace because "they can't focus in clutter." Some of these might be legitimate accommodations. But some might be you assuming responsibility that isn't yours.

You feel resentful but guilty about the resentment. You know you're doing too much. You're exhausted. But you also feel like you can't stop because your partner needs you. You're trapped between your needs and their limitations.

Your partner has stopped trying in certain areas. They've completely ceded responsibility for bills or schedules or household tasks. They don't even attempt these things because they know you'll handle them. This is learned helplessness, and it's not helping either of you.

You make excuses for your partner's behavior to others. When they forget plans with friends, you explain their AuDHD. When they're late to family events, you run interference. You've become their spokesperson and buffer against consequences.

Breaking codependency doesn't mean abandoning your partner. It means establishing healthy boundaries around what you will and won't do, building systems that allow them to be more independent, and accepting that they'll sometimes fail even with support. They need to experience natural consequences sometimes. You need to protect your own wellbeing and not sacrifice yourself on the altar of helpfulness.

Setting Boundaries Based on Strengths

Healthy division of household labor in neurodiverse relationships works differently than in neurotypical relationships. You can't just split everything 50/50. You need to divide responsibilities based on each person's actual capabilities and limitations.

Your partner might be terrible at consistent daily tasks but excellent at complex problem-solving. They can't remember to take out the trash every Tuesday, but they can troubleshoot the computer network or research the best cell phone plan. Assign them tasks that play to their strengths rather than forcing them to constantly perform in areas they struggle.

They might do better with variable tasks than routine ones. Their ADHD brain gets bored with repetition. So instead of assigning them the same chores every week, give them project-based responsibilities. They handle home repairs. You handle weekly cleaning. They manage one-time problem-solving. You manage recurring maintenance.

They might need tasks with clear deadlines and immediate consequences. They can't maintain ongoing systems, but they respond well to urgent needs. They're useless at regular car

41

maintenance but excellent in a crisis. Structure their responsibilities around this reality rather than fighting it.

Here's what this looks like practically: You might handle all bill payments and schedule management because those require consistency and time awareness. They handle all tech troubleshooting and research projects because those provide novelty and engage their hyperfocus. You manage the weekly grocery shopping because it requires routine. They handle meal planning because it requires creativity and variety.

This isn't "fair" in a traditional sense. You might handle more tasks. But fairness in neurodiverse relationships means each person contributes according to their abilities, not according to an arbitrary 50/50 split. You need to decide what matters more—theoretical equality or actual functionality.

Outsourcing: When External Systems Beat Internal Struggle

Sometimes the best solution is admitting that neither partner should handle certain tasks. Outsourcing isn't giving up or admitting failure. It's recognizing that some things work better when handled by external systems or people.

Automatic bill payments eliminate the need for either partner to remember due dates. Meal delivery services remove the executive function burden of meal planning and grocery shopping. Hiring a cleaning service once a month addresses the tasks neither partner can consistently maintain. Using a laundry service handles the folding your partner can't focus on and you don't have time for.

Yes, these solutions cost money. But the relationship costs of constant conflict over household tasks might be higher. You need to calculate the actual price of managing these things yourselves—not just financial cost but emotional toll, relationship damage, and time spent arguing about who didn't do what.

Your partner might resist outsourcing because it makes them feel like they're failing at basic adulting. They want to be capable of handling their own life. You might resist because it feels like you're being indulgent or wasteful. But if the alternative is ongoing resentment and conflict, outsourcing is a relationship investment, not an extravagance.

You can also outsource executive function support without outsourcing the tasks themselves. A body doubling service where someone works alongside your partner virtually can help them initiate and maintain focus on tasks. A virtual assistant can send reminders and check in on task completion. An ADHD coach can help develop systems and strategies. These supports acknowledge that your partner needs help without making you responsible for providing all that help.

Building Systems That Actually Work

Generic organization advice doesn't work for AuDHD brains. You need systems designed specifically for how their brain operates.

Visual reminders beat mental notes every time. Your partner won't remember things they can't see. Put bills to be paid in a visible spot, not filed away. Hang the calendar on the wall, don't keep it in a drawer. Use sticky notes, whiteboards, anything that keeps information in their visual field.

Timers are essential for time blindness. Your partner needs external time tracking because internal time tracking doesn't work. Set alarms for when to start getting ready. Use timers to limit time spent on tasks that tend to expand. Create alerts for transitions between activities.

Checklists compensate for working memory deficits. Your partner can't hold multi-step processes in their head. They need checklists for everything—morning routines, meal preparation, getting ready to leave the house. This isn't insulting. It's accommodating how their brain works.

Everything needs a home with clear labeling. Your partner loses things constantly because they don't have consistent places to put items. Create specific homes for frequently lost items and label them clearly. Keys go on this hook. Wallet goes in this basket. Phone charges in this spot. Remove the memory burden of "where did I put that?"

Break big projects into tiny chunks. Your partner can't tackle "clean the garage." They can handle "sort items in this box." Make tasks so small they seem ridiculously easy. That's the level of breakdown their executive function needs.

Use technology ruthlessly. Apps, alarms, automated systems—these are accommodations, not crutches. Your partner needs these tools the same way someone with poor vision needs glasses. Shared calendars, reminder apps, habit tracking apps, meditation timers, whatever helps their brain function better.

Build in flexibility and forgiveness. Systems that require perfect adherence will fail. Your partner's brain can't do perfect consistency. Build in margins for error. Allow tasks to shift by a day or two. Accept "good enough" instead of insisting on ideal execution.

The Follow-Up Email Trick

Here's a simple technique that prevents countless misunderstandings and forgotten agreements: after every important discussion, one partner sends a brief email or text summarizing what was decided and what each person agreed to do.

You have a conversation about vacation plans. Afterward, you text: "To confirm: we're going to Maine Aug 5-12, you'll book the cabin this week, I'll arrange pet care, we'll split the grocery planning." This creates a written record that compensates for your partner's working memory challenges.

You discuss a household issue. You send a follow-up email: "We agreed you'll handle the car maintenance this month and I'll tackle the yard work. The goal is to complete these by the end of next weekend. Let me know if you need any help getting started."

This isn't nagging or micromanaging. It's creating external memory support. Your partner can refer back to the summary when they inevitably forget details of the conversation. They have clear expectations in writing. You both have confirmation of what was agreed upon, which prevents later disagreements about "but I thought you said..."

Keep these summaries brief and factual. Don't editorialize or add passive-aggressive commentary. Just document the decisions and action items. This technique is especially helpful for complex plans or multi-step projects where details matter.

Resisting the Urge to Take Over

You'll be tempted to take over constantly. Your partner starts a task slowly and inefficiently. You could do it faster. You could do it better. You could save time by just handling it yourself. This impulse is the path to the parent-child dynamic. Resist it.

Let your partner struggle sometimes. Let them take three times as long as you would. Let them do things imperfectly. Unless the consequences are genuinely serious, give them space to figure things out their way.

Yes, watching them struggle is uncomfortable. Your instinct is to rescue. But rescuing reinforces their belief that they're incompetent and your belief that you have to manage everything. They need opportunities to succeed independently, even if success takes longer and looks messier than your version would.

You can offer help without taking over. "Do you want me to work alongside you?" is different from "Let me just do this." "I'm happy to help if you get stuck" is different from "You're doing it wrong, here's how." Make yourself available as support while respecting their agency to complete the task.

Sometimes your partner will ask you to take over. They're frustrated, overwhelmed, and want you to handle it. You need to discern between legitimate requests for help and requests that feed codependency. If taking over this one time helps them recover from being overwhelmed, fine. If taking over this one time continues a pattern of you managing their responsibilities, push back gently. "I believe you can handle this. What would help you get unstuck?"

What Success Actually Looks Like

Success in managing executive function challenges doesn't mean your partner suddenly becomes organized and punctual. Success means you've built systems that work well enough most of the time, you've divided responsibilities based on actual capabilities, and you've both accepted the limitations and found ways to work within them.

Your partner will still be late sometimes. They'll still forget things occasionally. They'll still abandon projects partway through. But the frequency decreases. The impact lessens. And most importantly, you stop taking it personally and they stop drowning in shame about it.

You'll still feel frustrated sometimes. Accommodating executive function deficits requires ongoing effort from you. But the frustration becomes manageable rather than constant. You understand what's happening and why, which reduces the emotional charge.

You both stop fighting against reality. You accept that your partner's brain works differently and build life around that reality rather than trying to force their brain to function neurotypically. They accept that they need external supports and stop feeling ashamed about using them.

The relationship becomes more collaborative and less adversarial. You're partners tackling shared challenges rather than a frustrated manager and an inadequate employee. You respect each other's contributions even when they look different from what you initially expected.

What's Coming Next

You've started building systems to support executive function. But what happens when those systems fail and emotions overflow? The next chapter addresses the most frightening aspect of AuDHD relationships for many partners—meltdowns, shutdowns, and the hair-trigger emotional reactivity that can make you feel like you're walking on eggshells. You'll learn what's actually happening neurologically during these episodes and how to respond in ways that help rather than escalate.

Essential Points to Remember

- Time blindness is a real neurological phenomenon where the brain can't accurately track or estimate time passing

- Executive function deficits affect planning, organizing, prioritizing, initiating tasks, and completing multi-step processes

- The parent-child dynamic develops when the neurotypical partner gradually takes over all management responsibilities

- Codependency in neurodiverse relationships often disguises itself as helpful support

- Dividing responsibilities based on each person's strengths rather than arbitrary equality creates functionality

- Outsourcing difficult tasks through automation, services, or external support is a legitimate accommodation strategy

- Effective systems for AuDHD brains include visual reminders, timers, checklists, consistent item locations, and tiny task breakdowns

- Following up important discussions with written summaries compensates for working memory challenges

- Resisting the urge to take over allows your partner to develop independence and maintains healthy relationship dynamics

- Success means functional systems that work most of the time, not perfect executive function performance

Chapter 5: When Emotions Overflow

Navigating Meltdowns, Shutdowns, and Rejection Sensitivity

The fight started over something small. You mentioned that your partner forgot to call your mother back. Just a simple observation. But your partner's face crumpled. Their eyes filled with tears. They yelled, "You think I'm useless! You hate me! I can't do anything right!" Then they stormed into the bedroom and slammed the door. You're standing in the living room, completely bewildered. All you said was they forgot a phone call. How did that become evidence you hate them?

This kind of emotional escalation happens so frequently in relationships with AuDHD individuals that many partners develop a constant low-level anxiety. You feel like you're walking through a minefield. Any comment might trigger an explosion. You start censoring yourself, carefully choosing words, avoiding topics that might cause upset. The relationship becomes defined by what you can't talk about rather than what you can. You're exhausted from managing someone else's emotions while suppressing your own needs. And you genuinely don't understand why everything feels like a crisis.

Why AuDHD Amplifies Emotional Intensity

Research shows that people with both autism and ADHD experience significantly more emotional dysregulation than people with either condition alone. This isn't just adding autism's emotional challenges to ADHD's emotional challenges. It's a multiplicative effect where the combination creates more severe difficulties than you'd expect.

Autistic individuals already process emotions intensely and struggle with emotional regulation. Their nervous systems respond more strongly to stimuli. They have difficulty modulating emotional responses to match the situation. A minor frustration feels catastrophic. A small disappointment triggers profound sadness.

ADHD adds impulsivity and reduced ability to pause between feeling and reacting. Neurotypical people have a small gap between emotional activation and emotional expression. You feel angry, then you decide how to express that anger. ADHD brains have a much smaller gap. They feel angry and the anger comes out immediately, often before they've consciously registered what they're feeling.

When you combine these factors in AuDHD, you get someone whose emotions are already running at high intensity and who lacks the ability to pause and regulate before reacting. They feel things more strongly than neurotypical people and have less ability to manage those feelings. The result is frequent emotional flooding, where they're completely overwhelmed by feelings they can't control.

Add in chronic stress from living in a neurotypical world that doesn't accommodate their needs, exhaustion from constant masking, shame from years of being told they're "too much," and anxiety about being rejected for their differences. Now you have someone operating at the edge of their regulatory capacity most of the time. Small stressors become the final straw that triggers emotional overflow.

Meltdowns vs. Shutdowns

Your partner's emotional overwhelm shows up in two distinct patterns: meltdowns and shutdowns. Both are responses to nervous system overload, but they look completely different on the outside.

Meltdowns are explosive. Your partner might yell, cry intensely, say things they don't mean, throw objects, storm out of rooms, or collapse sobbing. They might accuse you of things that aren't true. They might threaten to leave. They might describe catastrophic interpretations of situations. The emotional expression is loud, visible, and overwhelming for everyone involved.

Meltdowns aren't tantrums. Your partner isn't trying to manipulate you or punish you. They've lost the ability to regulate their emotional responses. The nervous system has hit overload and emergency protocols have kicked in. Their prefrontal cortex—the part of the brain that manages emotional regulation and rational thinking—has gone offline. They're in pure survival mode, driven by the emotional part of the brain with no access to the rational part.

Shutdowns are implosive. Your partner might go completely silent. They stop responding to questions. They can't make eye contact. They might stare blankly or leave the room without explanation. They seem to be physically present but mentally absent. Sometimes they literally can't speak—the ability to produce language temporarily disappears.

Shutdowns happen when the nervous system responds to overload by shutting down non-essential functions. Your partner's brain is protecting itself by reducing all input and output. They're not giving you the silent treatment or choosing to ignore you. They've lost the ability to process language, formulate responses, and engage socially. The shutdown is involuntary.

Both meltdowns and shutdowns are physiological responses to nervous system overload, not character flaws or deliberate choices. Your partner can't just "calm down" or "snap out of it" through willpower. Their nervous system needs time to regulate before they can regain access to their emotional regulation capacities.

Case Example 1: The Birthday Party Meltdown

Sophie had been planning her 30th birthday party for weeks. Her girlfriend Emma had helped with arrangements, and everything seemed set. The party was at a restaurant Sophie loved, with a small group of close friends. Emma felt good about how things were organized.

The night of the party, Emma wore a new dress Sophie hadn't seen before. When Sophie saw it, her face changed. She said quietly, "You look nice," but Emma could see something was wrong. The party proceeded, but Sophie seemed tense and distracted. Emma kept asking if she was okay. Sophie kept saying yes.

Halfway through dinner, Sophie suddenly stood up and announced she was leaving. Emma followed her outside, confused and concerned. Sophie started crying intensely. "You don't even care about me! You wore that dress to show me up on my birthday! You wanted everyone to look at you instead of me! I can't believe you'd be so selfish!"

Emma was stunned. She'd worn the dress because she wanted to look nice for Sophie's special day. She had no intention of upstaging anyone. She tried to explain this, but Sophie wouldn't hear it. She kept spiraling into more catastrophic interpretations. "This proves you don't love me. You want to humiliate me. I should have known better than to trust you."

Here's what actually happened: Sophie's autistic brain was already overwhelmed by the social demands of the party. She was masking heavily, managing anxiety about being the center of attention, and trying to ensure everyone was having a good time. When she saw Emma's beautiful dress, her ADHD brain made an impulsive connection: "She looks better than me, people will pay attention to her instead of me, this party isn't about me anymore." This thought triggered anxiety, which triggered more catastrophic thoughts, which built into emotional flooding.

Sophie's rational brain knew Emma hadn't done anything wrong. But her rational brain wasn't accessible. She was operating from pure emotional reactivity. The meltdown wasn't about the dress. The dress was the trigger that released accumulated stress that had been building all week.

Emma didn't understand this at the time. She felt attacked and blamed for something she didn't do. The party ended early. Their friends were confused. Emma felt embarrassed and angry. Sophie felt ashamed and misunderstood.

Later, after Sophie had time to regulate, she could recognize what happened. She apologized. She explained the stress buildup and how the dress became the breaking point. Emma could see how the meltdown wasn't really about her actions. But in the moment, it felt like an unfair attack.

They developed a better system. Before big events, Sophie now tells Emma her stress level. If she's already close to capacity, they make plans to reduce additional stressors. Sophie also worked on recognizing earlier warning signs of approaching meltdown so she could take breaks before completely losing regulation.

Case Example 2: The Grocery Store Shutdown

Marcus and his partner Trent were shopping together on a Saturday afternoon. The store was crowded and loud. They'd been there about 20 minutes when Marcus noticed Trent had stopped talking. He was staring blankly at the shelf, not moving.

"Which pasta sauce do you want?" Marcus asked. No response. "Trent? Hello?" Still nothing. Trent's eyes were open but he wasn't reacting to anything Marcus said. Marcus felt a flash of anger. Was Trent seriously ignoring him over pasta sauce?

He tried again, more forcefully. "Trent, I'm talking to you!" Nothing. Marcus waved his hand in front of Trent's face. Trent blinked but didn't speak. Marcus felt frustrated and concerned in equal measure. He didn't know if Trent was upset with him, having some kind of medical episode, or what.

Marcus finished the shopping quickly and guided Trent to the car. Trent moved mechanically, following directions but not speaking. In the car, he stared out the window silently. At home, he went directly to the bedroom, closed the door, and stayed there for three hours.

Marcus was hurt and confused. What had he done wrong? Why was Trent shutting him out? When Trent finally emerged, he looked exhausted. Marcus asked what happened. Trent explained he'd experienced a shutdown.

The sensory input in the crowded store had been overwhelming. The bright lights, loud sounds, competing conversations, and constant movement overloaded Trent's autistic sensory processing. His ADHD meant he couldn't filter out the irrelevant stimuli—everything demanded equal attention. Combined stress from work earlier that week and poor sleep had left him with minimal regulatory capacity. The grocery store pushed him past his limit.

During the shutdown, Trent physically couldn't speak. The ability to produce language disappeared. He could hear Marcus but couldn't process the words or formulate responses. His brain had shut down all non-essential functions. He wasn't choosing to ignore Marcus. He literally couldn't respond.

Marcus had interpreted the shutdown as deliberate ignoring or passive-aggressive punishment. Now he understood it was an involuntary neurological response. They created a signal system. When Trent feels a shutdown approaching, he taps Marcus's arm three times. This tells Marcus that Trent is getting overwhelmed and they need to leave or find a quiet space. They also avoid shopping at peak times and limit trip duration to prevent future shutdowns.

Case Example 3: The Work Feedback Spiral

Jordan's partner Alex worked in software development. One day, Alex's manager gave feedback on a project. The feedback was mild and constructive—just suggestions for improving the code structure. But when Alex came home, they were devastated.

"I'm getting fired," Alex announced. "My manager hates me. I'm terrible at this job. I should just quit before they fire me. I'm such a failure." Jordan was confused. Alex had shown them the actual feedback email, and it seemed perfectly reasonable and supportive. Jordan tried to point this out.

"Your manager said you're doing well overall. They just suggested some improvements. That's normal feedback." But Alex couldn't hear this. They spiraled deeper into catastrophic thinking. "You don't understand. This means I'm incompetent. They're disappointed in me. They're just being nice because they're building a case to fire me later."

This went on for hours. Alex couldn't be reassured or reasoned with. They were certain they were about to lose their job despite zero evidence supporting this belief. Jordan felt helpless and frustrated. How could one piece of minor feedback trigger such an extreme reaction?

Alex was experiencing Rejection Sensitive Dysphoria (RSD), a condition common in ADHD where perceived criticism or rejection triggers overwhelming emotional pain. The manager's feedback, which was intended as helpful guidance, was processed by Alex's brain as devastating rejection. The rational assessment ("this is normal feedback") couldn't override the emotional experience ("I'm being rejected and I'm worthless").

The ADHD lens distorted the manager's words. "This code structure could be improved" became "You're a bad developer." "Consider this alternative approach" became "Your approach was wrong." Alex's brain translated neutral, constructive feedback into evidence of personal failure.

Alex also struggled with shame accumulated from years of making mistakes, forgetting things, and being criticized for ADHD symptoms. Any new criticism felt like confirmation of deeply held fears about being inadequate. The emotional response wasn't proportionate to the actual feedback. It was proportionate to all the accumulated shame and fear of rejection.

Jordan learned that arguing with Alex during RSD spirals didn't help. Alex couldn't access rational thinking when emotionally flooded. Instead, Jordan started acknowledging the pain without trying to fix or argue with Alex's interpretation. "This feels really scary for you right now. I hear that you're hurting." Over time, as the emotional intensity decreased, Alex could gradually reconnect with rational assessment of the situation.

They also implemented a waiting period. When Alex received any feedback, they agreed to wait 24 hours before making any decisions about what it meant. This gave the emotional response time to settle and allowed Alex to process the feedback more rationally later.

Understanding Rejection Sensitive Dysphoria

RSD deserves special attention because it creates so much relationship conflict. Your partner doesn't just feel hurt by criticism. They feel emotionally devastated. The pain is physical and overwhelming. They describe it as feeling like they're dying or being stabbed. Small criticisms feel like existential threats.

This means you genuinely can't have certain conversations without triggering severe emotional reactions. You can't offer constructive feedback the way you would with a neurotypical partner. You can't point out problems directly. You can't express disappointment without your partner interpreting it as complete rejection.

Your partner probably knows their reaction is disproportionate. After they calm down, they can recognize that your comment wasn't devastating. But in the moment, their brain interprets any hint of criticism or rejection as catastrophic. They can't control this response any more than someone can control a panic attack.

RSD is particularly triggered by feedback from people they care about. Criticism from you hurts more than criticism from strangers because rejection by you matters more. This creates a terrible dynamic where the person whose opinion matters most is also the person whose feedback triggers the most intense pain.

Your partner might also experience RSD around perceived rejection. You didn't text back quickly, so clearly you're angry with them. You seemed distracted during a conversation, so obviously you don't care about them anymore. You made plans with friends, so you must be pulling away from the relationship. These interpretations feel absolutely true to them, even when they're objectively false.

The Constant Self-Explanation Trap

Many neurodivergent individuals in relationships with neurotypical partners feel like they're constantly explaining themselves. You ask why they did something a certain way. They have to explain their ADHD made them lose focus. You express concern about a behavior. They have to explain their autism makes social situations stressful. You wonder why they seem upset. They have to explain their sensory sensitivity was triggered.

This creates exhausting hypervigilance. Your partner is constantly monitoring themselves, anticipating your questions or concerns, preparing explanations for behaviors they know might seem odd. They're defending their neurological differences over and over. This builds shame and guilt. They start to feel like they're fundamentally broken and constantly burdening you with their problems.

You might not realize you're creating this dynamic. You're just trying to understand your partner better. But from their perspective, every question feels like an accusation they have to defend against. Every expression of concern feels like evidence they're too difficult to love.

This pattern also shows up around boundaries. Your partner says no to something. You ask why. They explain their capacity is low. You push back with solutions that would make it possible. They have to explain again why their no stands. You keep problem-solving. They keep explaining. Eventually they feel like their boundaries aren't respected and you feel like they're not willing to compromise.

Breaking this pattern requires you to accept no without requiring justification. Your partner says they can't attend a social event. You accept this without demanding an explanation or offering solutions. They say they need alone time. You respect that

58

without making them explain why or how long. They decline to do something. You trust their self-assessment without interrogating it.

Your partner isn't being difficult. They're managing limitations you can't see. Requiring constant explanation makes those limitations feel shameful rather than neutral facts about how their brain works.

What to Do During a Meltdown

Your instinct during your partner's meltdown is to fix it, calm them down, or reason with them. None of this works. You can't logic someone out of an emotional state that's bypassed their logical brain. Here's what actually helps:

Create physical and emotional safety. Remove immediate dangers. If they're breaking things, gently guide them away from breakables. If they're in a public space, help them get somewhere private. Your priority is preventing harm, not stopping the meltdown.

Reduce sensory input. Dim lights, reduce noise, minimize activity around them. Their nervous system is already overloaded. Additional stimulation makes it worse. Create a calm environment that helps their system settle.

Give them space without abandoning them. Your partner needs room to experience the meltdown without feeling crowded or pressured. But they also need to know you're not leaving. You might say, "I'm going to step into the other room. I'll be here when you're ready." This gives them space while providing security.

Don't argue with what they're saying. During meltdowns, your partner might say hurtful, untrue, catastrophic things. They might accuse you of not loving them, claim the relationship is over, or express distorted interpretations of situations. Don't defend yourself or correct these statements in the moment. Their emotional brain is in charge and it's not processing rational information.

Wait for regulation before discussing anything. You can't resolve issues or clarify misunderstandings during a meltdown. Their prefrontal cortex is offline. Wait until they've calmed completely before attempting any conversation about what happened or what triggered it.

Have a plan you've created together. Talk with your partner when they're calm about what helps during meltdowns. Do they want you nearby or away? Do they want physical touch or no touch? Do they want you to talk to them or stay silent? Everyone's different. Create a plan specific to your partner's needs.

What NOT to Do During a Meltdown

Don't tell them to calm down. This is useless and makes things worse. They would calm down if they could. Telling them to do something they're currently incapable of doing adds frustration and shame.

Don't touch them without permission. Unsolicited touch during emotional overwhelm can trigger more distress. Some people find touch soothing. Others find it intolerable. Know your partner's preference and respect it.

Don't take what they say personally. Your partner is not expressing considered thoughts. They're in emotional flooding. The things they say during meltdowns often don't reflect their actual beliefs. They're the emotional brain's panic responses, not the thinking brain's assessments.

Don't try to problem-solve. "Let's figure out what triggered this" or "Here's what you should do next time" are conversations for later. Right now, their brain can't access problem-solving capacity. Save those discussions for when they've recovered.

Don't punish or withdraw affection. Meltdowns are not behavior problems requiring discipline. They're neurological events. Your partner already feels ashamed. Punishment or withdrawal adds to that shame and damages trust.

Don't bring up old issues or continue the triggering conversation. The meltdown paused whatever you were discussing. Don't try to resume it. That discussion needs to wait until your partner has fully regulated, and it might need to happen in a completely different way.

What to Do During a Shutdown

Shutdowns require different responses than meltdowns because your partner's needs are different.

Recognize it's a shutdown, not silent treatment. Your partner isn't choosing to ignore you. They've temporarily lost the ability to process and produce language. This distinction matters because it changes how you respond.

Stop requiring verbal communication. Don't keep asking questions they can't answer. Don't expect conversation. Accept that verbal communication is temporarily unavailable.

Minimize demands and decisions. Your partner can't handle additional cognitive load during a shutdown. Don't ask them to make decisions or complete tasks. Reduce demands to absolute minimum.

Create a quiet space. Help them get somewhere with low sensory input where they can rest without stimulation. Their nervous system needs calm to reset.

Give them time without pressure. Shutdowns last as long as they last. You can't rush the process. Your partner needs to rest until their nervous system recovers the ability to engage. This might take minutes, hours, or longer.

Offer simple options without requiring response. "I'm going to get you some water and a blanket" is better than "Do you want water? What about a blanket? Are you cold? Should I..." Provide basic comfort without demanding interaction.

Creating a Prevention Plan

The best way to handle meltdowns and shutdowns is preventing them when possible. This requires your partner to recognize their warning signs and both of you to have a plan for reducing stress before they hit complete overload.

Identify early warning signs together. When your partner is calm, discuss what they notice before meltdowns or shutdowns. Do they feel increasingly irritable? Do they become quieter? Do they start feeling overwhelmed by sensory input? Do they notice physical tension? Create a list of personal warning signs.

Establish a signal system. Your partner needs a way to communicate "I'm approaching my limit" before they lose the ability to communicate. This might be a specific word, a hand gesture, or a text with a predetermined code. When you receive this signal, you know they need support before reaching crisis.

Make an inventory of common triggers. What situations, conversations, or experiences frequently lead to emotional overwhelm for your partner? Crowded spaces? Certain types of feedback? Schedule disruptions? Relationship conflict? Financial stress? Knowing triggers helps you both avoid or prepare for high-risk situations.

Build in recovery time. Schedule downtime after stressful events. Your partner's regulatory capacity is limited and gets depleted. They need protected time to recharge before they're completely empty. If they have a stressful work week, don't plan big social events for the weekend. If they have a difficult family gathering, give them quiet time afterward.

Create a written plan. Document what helps during meltdowns and shutdowns. What do they need from you? What makes things worse? What helps them recover afterward? Having this written down means you don't have to remember everything in the moment and your partner doesn't have to explain while overwhelmed.

Supporting Without Enabling

You want to help your partner manage emotional regulation challenges. But you also don't want to become responsible for managing their emotions for them or preventing all distress. The line between support and enabling can be blurry.

Support looks like: Recognizing warning signs and suggesting breaks. Creating a calm environment during recovery. Respecting their communication needs. Validating their emotional experience without agreeing with distorted interpretations. Helping them identify patterns and triggers.

Enabling looks like: Walking on eggshells to prevent any upset. Taking responsibility for their emotional state. Censoring all your needs and feelings to avoid triggering them. Making excuses for their behavior to others. Organizing your entire life around preventing their meltdowns.

You can acknowledge your partner's pain without agreeing their catastrophic interpretation is accurate. "I can see you're really hurt right now" is different from "You're right, I clearly don't care about you." You validate the emotion without reinforcing the distortion.

You can provide space for recovery without abandoning your own needs indefinitely. After a meltdown, your partner might need several hours alone. That's fine. But you also get to say, "I need us to discuss what happened within the next day or two because I have feelings about this too." You accommodate their recovery needs while maintaining that your feelings also matter.

You can help them recognize patterns without becoming their emotional monitor. "I've noticed you tend to have meltdowns on Sunday evenings. I wonder if the stress of the upcoming work week contributes?" This opens awareness without making it your job to prevent Sunday evening meltdowns forever.

Your partner is responsible for learning their patterns, developing coping strategies, and working on emotional regulation skills over time. You can support this work. You cannot do it for them.

Looking Forward

Managing emotional intensity is exhausting for both partners. You're constantly navigating triggers, responding to overwhelm, and managing the aftermath of meltdowns and shutdowns. But there's another layer to this challenge. The next chapter addresses sensory processing—the invisible world of stimuli that constantly bombards your partner's nervous system and contributes heavily to the emotional overwhelm you're managing. Understanding sensory differences helps prevent many of the emotional crises this chapter addressed.

Critical Lessons for Partners

- AuDHD creates more severe emotional dysregulation than autism or ADHD alone through multiplicative effects on emotional intensity and impulse control

- Meltdowns are explosive nervous system overload responses, not tantrums or manipulation attempts

- Shutdowns involve temporary loss of language processing and production abilities, not deliberate silent treatment

- Rejection Sensitive Dysphoria causes disproportionate emotional pain in response to criticism or perceived rejection

- Constant demands for self-explanation create hypervigilance, shame, and exhaustion in neurodivergent partners

- During meltdowns, create safety, reduce sensory input, and provide space without abandoning your partner

- During shutdowns, eliminate communication demands, minimize decisions, and allow recovery time without pressure

- Prevention plans should identify warning signs, establish signal systems, document triggers, and outline helpful responses

- Support involves validating emotions and accommodating recovery needs while maintaining your own boundaries and needs

- Your partner is responsible for developing emotional regulation skills over time, not you

Chapter 6: The Sensory World You Can't See

Understanding and Accommodating Their Unique Nervous System

You planned a romantic evening at that new restaurant everyone raves about. The food is supposed to be amazing. You got reservations. You're excited. But within ten minutes of arriving, your partner looks miserable. They're sitting rigidly, not making eye contact, giving one-word answers. They pick at their food. They say they're fine but clearly aren't. Later, they might explain they couldn't focus on anything because the music was too loud, the lights were too bright, their shirt tag was itching, and the smell from the kitchen was overwhelming. To you, these were background details—barely noticeable. To them, these sensory inputs were screaming for attention, making it impossible to think, converse, or enjoy anything. The romantic evening you planned became an endurance test they had to survive.

Sensory processing differences are invisible but powerful. You can't see your partner's nervous system responding to stimuli you barely notice. You can't feel their physical pain from sounds you find pleasant. You can't experience their overwhelming distress from textures you don't even register. This creates a gap where your partner seems to be overreacting to nothing while actually managing what feels to them like physical assault from their environment.

Why AuDHD Makes Sensory Processing More Challenging

Research shows that people with both autism and ADHD have significantly more sensory processing differences than people with either condition alone. The combination creates unique challenges.

Autistic individuals typically process sensory information more intensely. Their nervous systems are more sensitive to input. Sounds are louder. Lights are brighter. Textures are more noticeable. Smells are stronger. This isn't psychological—it's neurological. Their sensory system has lower thresholds and stronger responses.

ADHD adds a different problem: difficulty filtering sensory input. Neurotypical brains automatically filter out irrelevant stimuli. You can have a conversation in a noisy restaurant because your brain screens out the background noise and focuses on the person speaking. ADHD brains struggle with this filtering. Everything demands equal attention. The background music, neighboring conversations, kitchen sounds, and the person speaking all compete equally for processing resources.

When you combine autism's intensity with ADHD's inability to filter, you get someone whose nervous system is bombarded by intense stimuli they can't ignore. They're experiencing everything at high volume with no capacity to tune out the irrelevant parts. This is exhausting and overwhelming even in environments you find perfectly comfortable.

AuDHD individuals often experience sensory overload more frequently and more severely than people with just autism or just ADHD. The combination creates a lower threshold for overwhelm and longer recovery periods afterward.

The Eight Sensory Systems

Most people think of five senses: sight, hearing, touch, taste, and smell. But there are actually eight sensory systems that can be affected in AuDHD individuals. Understanding all eight helps you recognize sensory triggers you might be missing.

Visual processing involves how the brain handles what the eyes see. Your partner might be hypersensitive to bright lights, fluorescent lighting, screens, or busy patterns. They might find certain colors physically painful to look at. Or they might be hyposensitive and seek out visual stimulation through screens, spinning objects, or watching moving things.

Auditory processing involves sounds. Your partner might be hypersensitive to volume, certain frequencies, overlapping sounds, or unexpected noises. Background music that you barely notice might feel painfully loud to them. Or they might be hyposensitive and need louder volume or constant background noise to feel comfortable.

Tactile processing involves touch and texture. Your partner might be hypersensitive to certain fabrics, tags in clothing, light touches, or unexpected contact. They might find hugs painful or certain textures intolerable. Or they might be hyposensitive and seek out deep pressure, tight clothing, or specific textures.

Gustatory processing involves taste. Your partner might be hypersensitive to certain flavors, textures of food, or temperatures. They might have a very limited diet because most foods feel unbearable in their mouth. Or they might be hyposensitive and seek out strong flavors or unusual food combinations.

Olfactory processing involves smell. Your partner might be hypersensitive to perfumes, food smells, cleaning products, or body odors. Scents you don't even notice might cause them physical nausea or headaches. Or they might be hyposensitive and not notice smells that other people find obvious.

Vestibular processing involves balance and movement. Your partner might be hypersensitive to motion, get dizzy easily, or feel disoriented by certain movements. Or they might be hyposensitive and seek out spinning, swinging, or intense movement experiences.

Proprioceptive processing involves body awareness and position. Your partner might be hypersensitive and feel overwhelmed by physical contact or movement. Or they might be hyposensitive and seek out deep pressure, tight hugs, or heavy blankets because they struggle to feel where their body is in space without intense input.

Interoceptive processing involves internal body sensations like hunger, thirst, temperature, pain, and need to use the bathroom. Your partner might struggle to recognize these signals until they're extreme. They might not realize they're hungry until they're dizzy or not notice they're cold until they're shivering.

Most people are a mix—hypersensitive in some systems and hyposensitive in others. Your partner might be overwhelmed by sounds but seek out intense visual input. They might hate being touched lightly but crave deep pressure. Understanding their specific sensory profile helps you accommodate their needs.

Case Example 1: The Shopping Mall Shutdown

Teresa and her boyfriend Michael went to the mall on a Saturday afternoon. Michael needed to return something at one store, then wanted to browse a few others. Teresa had been quiet in the car but agreed to come along. Thirty minutes into the trip, she said she needed to leave immediately. Michael was confused—they'd barely started. Teresa was insistent. They had to go now.

In the car, Teresa looked exhausted and on the verge of tears. Michael asked what happened. Teresa tried to explain but struggled to find words. Eventually she described a cascade of sensory assault: the fluorescent lighting was physically painful, creating headaches and making it hard to focus visually. The competing sounds—music from different stores, announcements, crowds of people talking, children crying—all demanded her attention simultaneously. She couldn't filter any of it out. Her clothes felt wrong—the waistband was too tight, the shirt fabric was itchy. Too many people were too close to her body in crowded areas. The mix of perfumes, food court smells, and cleaning products made her nauseated.

Each of these inputs alone would have been manageable for a short time. Combined, they created overwhelming sensory overload. Teresa tried to endure it because she knew Michael wanted to shop. But her nervous system reached capacity. She had to escape before experiencing a complete shutdown or meltdown in public.

Michael was surprised. He'd found the mall perfectly comfortable. Sure, it was busy, but that was normal for Saturday. He didn't realize Teresa was experiencing the same environment completely differently. To him, the sounds were background noise. To her, they were individual assault. To him, the crowds were slightly annoying. To her, they were painful invasion of her personal space. Same physical environment, radically different neurological experience.

They changed their approach. Now Michael shops alone or during off-peak hours when the mall is quieter. When they do go together, they plan short trips with clear time limits and have an escape plan Teresa can initiate anytime. They also identify quiet spots in the mall where Teresa can take sensory breaks. These accommodations allow Teresa to sometimes accompany Michael without sacrificing her nervous system in the process.

Case Example 2: The Intimacy Disconnect

Luis and his wife Jenna had been married for three years. Their physical intimacy had steadily decreased, and Luis felt hurt and confused. Jenna seemed to avoid physical contact. She'd pull away from hugs. She rarely initiated intimate touch. During sex, she seemed distracted and uncomfortable, though she insisted she wanted to be close to him.

Luis started to believe Jenna wasn't attracted to him anymore. Jenna felt guilty and frustrated. She did want physical closeness with Luis. But so many aspects of physical intimacy triggered sensory sensitivities that she spent the entire experience managing discomfort rather than connecting with her partner.

When they finally had an honest conversation, Jenna explained her sensory experience: light touch felt like irritation rather than pleasure, triggering a reflexive pull-away response. Certain touches triggered overwhelm rather than arousal. The sounds Luis made during intimacy, which were natural expressions, sometimes felt too loud or too close to her ears. Scented products like lotions, cologne, or even laundry detergent on the sheets were distracting or unpleasant. The bedroom lighting was often too bright. Temperature changes during intimacy left her uncomfortable—too hot or too cold. Oral sensitivities meant certain types of kissing felt intolerable rather than intimate.

None of this meant Jenna didn't love Luis or wasn't attracted to him. It meant her sensory system processed physical intimacy very differently than his did. What felt good to him didn't necessarily feel good to her. What he didn't even notice—the detergent smell, the light level, the specific type of touch—her brain processed as significant sensory input that competed with ability to be present and connected.

They rebuilt their physical intimacy around Jenna's sensory needs. They experimented with different types of touch to identify what felt pleasant to her rather than just assuming neurotypical touch preferences would work. They adjusted bedroom environment—lighting, temperature, scents, fabrics. They established communication signals so Jenna could indicate "more of this" or "less of that" without having to verbally explain during intimate moments, which added cognitive load she couldn't manage while also trying to be present physically.

Luis had to release expectations about what physical intimacy "should" look like and learn what worked for Jenna's actual nervous system. Jenna had to communicate her needs clearly instead of trying to endure sensory discomfort to please Luis. Together they created intimacy patterns that worked for both of them.

Case Example 3: The Dinner Party Disaster

Priya invited her girlfriend Sara to a dinner party at a colleague's house. Priya was excited—this was a good networking opportunity and she wanted Sara there. Sara agreed hesitantly. She'd never been to this person's home before and didn't know what to expect sensorially.

They arrived and Priya immediately started mingling. Sara tried to engage but struggled. The dining room had bright overhead lighting with no dimmer. The host was burning a strong-scented candle. Multiple conversations happened simultaneously in a small space, creating overlapping noise. The furniture fabric felt scratchy and unpleasant. Dinner included several foods with textures Sara found intolerable—mushy vegetables, slimy sauces.

Sara tried to manage. She sat in the corner to reduce visual and auditory input. She quietly avoided foods she couldn't handle. But she was visibly struggling. Priya kept checking on her with concern that made Sara feel more stressed. After two hours, Sara whispered that she needed to leave. Priya was disappointed but agreed.

In the car, Priya expressed frustration. "You knew this was important to me. Couldn't you have tried a little harder?" Sara felt defensive and hurt. She *had* tried. She'd pushed through significant sensory discomfort for two hours. Priya thought Sara was being difficult or antisocial. Sara thought Priya didn't understand or care about her limitations.

This conflict stemmed from invisible sensory differences. Priya experienced the party as pleasantly stimulating. Sara experienced it as sensory assault. Priya saw Sara as not trying. Sara saw herself as enduring beyond her capacity. Neither could truly understand the other's experience.

They had to build better systems. Before accepting social invitations involving new environments, Sara needed more information: What's the lighting like? Will there be strong scents? How many people? How loud? How long? What food will be served? This allowed Sara to assess whether she could manage the sensory environment and prepare appropriately.

Priya had to accept that some events simply wouldn't work for Sara sensorially, and that wasn't personal rejection of Priya or the hosts. Sara had to communicate her needs more clearly upfront rather than agreeing to things and then struggling. They also established exit strategies—Sara could signal she needed to leave, and Priya would wrap up quickly without making Sara feel guilty or difficult.

Why "Small Things" Create Big Reactions

You might wonder why your partner can't just ignore sensory irritations the way you do. You hear the music and tune it out. They hear the music and can't stop noticing it. You feel the shirt tag and forget about it. They feel the shirt tag and it demands constant attention. Why can't they just redirect their focus?

The answer is neurological, not willpower. Your brain automatically filters sensory input, pushing irrelevant stimuli to the background. Their brain lacks this automatic filtering. Everything stays in foreground, demanding processing resources. They're constantly expending conscious effort to try to ignore sensations that your brain handles automatically.

Think of it like having 20 browser tabs open on your computer. Each tab uses processing power. Too many tabs slow everything down. Your partner's sensory experience is like having 50 tabs open while you have 5. They're trying to function while their system is overloaded with competing demands for attention.

Sensory input also accumulates. One sensory irritation is manageable. But bright lights *plus* scratchy clothing *plus* background noise *plus* strong smells equals overload. By the time you notice your partner is struggling, they've already been managing multiple sensory assaults for a while. What looks like sudden overreaction is actually the result of steady accumulation.

Sensory processing also drains regulatory capacity. Your partner is using mental energy just to exist in environments you find comfortable. By the time they need to regulate emotions, solve problems, or make decisions, they've already spent much of their available capacity on managing sensory input. This is why they might seem to have shorter fuses or less patience than neurotypical people—they're constantly operating at reduced capacity.

Creating Sensory-Friendly Home Environments

Your home should be a sensory refuge, not another environment your partner has to endure. You can't control the outside world, but you can control your shared living space. Here's how:

Lighting matters more than you think. Overhead fluorescent lighting is particularly problematic for many AuDHD individuals. Switch to lamps with warm bulbs. Install dimmers. Use string lights or other soft lighting options. Give your partner control over lighting levels in spaces they use frequently.

Sound management is critical. White noise machines or fans can mask unpredictable sounds that trigger startle responses. Good windows reduce external noise. Noise-canceling headphones or earplugs should be readily available. Accept that your partner might wear headphones at home frequently—this isn't rejection, it's sensory management.

Temperature control prevents constant discomfort. AuDHD individuals often have trouble regulating body temperature or are hypersensitive to temperature changes. Make sure your partner can easily adjust temperature in their spaces. Accept that they might wear layers indoors or want the temperature different than you prefer. This isn't them being difficult—their nervous system genuinely needs different conditions.

Scent awareness prevents invisible assault. Switch to unscented cleaning products, laundry detergents, and personal care items. Avoid air fresheners, candles, and strong perfumes in shared spaces. What smells pleasant to you might cause physical nausea or headaches for them.

Texture choices affect daily comfort. Let your partner choose their own clothing without judgment about what looks appropriate. If they wear the same comfortable outfit repeatedly, that's a sensory accommodation, not laziness. Choose furniture and bedding based on texture comfort, not just appearance. Soft fabrics, specific materials, or certain thread counts might make a significant difference.

Designate a low-sensory retreat space. Your partner needs somewhere to decompress when overwhelmed. This might be a bedroom, a corner with a comfortable chair, or any space that can be dimmed, quieted, and controlled. Respect this space as their sensory refuge.

Create predictability where possible. Unexpected sensory inputs are harder to manage than predictable ones. Warn your partner before using loud appliances, cooking strong-smelling foods, or making changes to the home environment. This allows them to prepare or leave the area temporarily.

Navigating Physical Intimacy Around Sensory Needs

Physical intimacy involves intense sensory input across multiple systems. This creates unique challenges that many couples struggle to discuss openly.

Have explicit conversations about touch preferences. Don't assume your partner likes what previous partners liked or what media portrays as pleasurable. Their sensory system might experience touch completely differently. Ask specifically what types of touch feel good, neutral, or bad. Light touch versus deep pressure. Different body areas. Different contexts.

Environment matters as much as actions. Bedroom lighting, temperature, sounds, smells, bedding texture—all impact your partner's ability to be present and comfortable. Optimize the environment before expecting them to relax and connect.

Communication needs to be non-verbal sometimes. Stopping to verbally explain sensory issues adds cognitive load. Develop signals—hand placement, specific words, gestures—that communicate "more," "less," "different," or "stop" without requiring full sentences and explanations.

Sensory sensitivities fluctuate. Something that felt fine last week might be intolerable today. Your partner's capacity changes based on stress, fatigue, hormones, and recent sensory overload. Don't take it personally when something that previously worked suddenly doesn't. Accept that flexibility is required.

Post-intimacy care includes sensory recovery. Your partner might need to decompress alone after physical intimacy to recover from sensory input. This isn't rejection. It's nervous system regulation. Respect this need without making them feel guilty for needing space.

Dating and Social Life With Sensory Limitations

Typical dating and social environments are often sensory nightmares: loud bars, crowded restaurants, bright clubs, strong-smelling venues. Your partner's limitations might feel like they're restricting your social life. This is a valid source of frustration, but it requires reframing.

Choose sensory-friendly venues. Quiet restaurants during off-peak hours. Outdoor spaces. Museums. Walks in nature. Coffee shops with good acoustics. These locations allow your partner to be present and engaged instead of just enduring.

Time social activities strategically. Your partner has limited capacity. Don't schedule multiple social events back-to-back or after a demanding work week. Give them recovery time before and after high-sensory situations.

Have an exit strategy. Your partner needs to know they can leave if sensory overload hits. Agree in advance on signals and procedures. This reduces anxiety about being trapped in intolerable situations.

Accept that some activities won't work. Concerts, festivals, crowded sporting events, busy nightlife venues—these might simply be incompatible with your partner's sensory system. You'll need to decide what's non-negotiable for you and where you're willing to compromise.

Attend events separately sometimes. You can go to loud concerts with friends while your partner stays home. They're not preventing you from doing these things. They're preventing you from doing them together. This might feel disappointing, but it's better than forcing your partner into situations that cause them genuine distress.

The Sensory-Emotion Connection

Sensory overload directly contributes to the emotional dysregulation you read about in the previous chapter. When your partner's nervous system is managing constant sensory assault, their capacity for emotional regulation disappears. They're already at maximum capacity just processing environmental input. Add an emotional stressor, and they've got nothing left.

This means sensory accommodation is emotional regulation support. When you reduce sensory demands on your partner, you're not just making them more comfortable—you're preserving their capacity to manage emotions, communicate effectively, and be present in the relationship.

Many meltdowns are actually sensory meltdowns triggered by accumulated sensory stress. The fight you had wasn't really about dishes. It was about dishes becoming the final stressor after your partner spent all day managing sensory input at work, dealt with traffic noise on the commute, and came home to bright lighting and strong cooking smells. The dishes were just the trigger that released pressure that had been building all day.

Understanding this connection helps you see patterns. Your partner tends to have meltdowns after spending time in certain places. They seem "touchy" after busy weekends. They withdraw after social events. These aren't random emotional problems—they're predictable responses to sensory overload.

You can prevent many emotional crises by managing sensory input proactively. Your partner comes home after a stressful day? Dim the lights, reduce noise, give them quiet time before expecting conversation. You're planning a busy weekend? Build in sensory recovery time. You notice warning signs of sensory overload? Help them exit the situation before it becomes emotional overflow.

What You Need from This

Your partner's sensory needs might feel like constant constraints on your life. You can't go certain places. You have to manage lighting, sound, and smells carefully. You're always checking if environments will work for them. This is legitimately limiting.

You're allowed to grieve the spontaneity and flexibility you thought your relationship would have. You're allowed to feel frustrated sometimes. You're allowed to miss activities you can't do together. These feelings don't make you unsupportive. They make you human.

But you also need to accept that your partner's sensory system works differently than yours, and this isn't going to change. No amount of exposure therapy or "getting used to it" will make their nervous system process input like yours does. Accommodations aren't temporary adjustments until they develop more tolerance. These are permanent needs based on neurological differences.

The question isn't how to make your partner's sensory sensitivities go away. The question is how to build a life together that accommodates both your needs. Sometimes this means you do things separately. Sometimes it means choosing different venues. Sometimes it means one person compromises more in certain areas while the other compromises more in different areas.

Your needs matter too. You might need a partner who can attend loud social events with you. You might need someone who can handle spontaneous plans. You might need a certain level of physical intimacy. If your partner genuinely can't meet these needs, you need to decide if the relationship can work. That's not cruel—it's honest assessment of compatibility.

Where We Go from Here

You've now learned about the three major challenges in AuDHD relationships: executive function deficits, emotional regulation struggles, and sensory processing differences. These create the daily frustrations and conflicts that make you question the relationship. But understanding them allows you to stop personalizing behaviors that aren't about you and start building systems that work for both of you.

The remaining chapters address how to identify and recover from burnout, how to fight constructively, how to maintain your own wellbeing while supporting your partner, and how to build a thriving relationship that celebrates your differences rather than being destroyed by them.

What You've Learned Here

- AuDHD creates more significant sensory processing differences than autism or ADHD alone through combined intensity and inability to filter input

- Eight sensory systems can be affected: visual, auditory, tactile, gustatory, olfactory, vestibular, proprioceptive, and interoceptive

- Individuals can be hypersensitive in some systems and hyposensitive in others, creating unique sensory profiles

- Sensory input accumulates throughout the day, leading to overload that appears as sudden emotional reactions

- Home environments should prioritize sensory accommodation through lighting, sound management, temperature control, scent awareness, and texture choices

- Physical intimacy requires explicit communication about touch preferences, environmental optimization, and non-verbal signaling systems

- Typical dating and social venues often create sensory assault that prevents connection and engagement

- Sensory overload directly reduces capacity for emotional regulation, contributing to meltdowns and irritability

- Partners need to accept sensory accommodations as permanent neurological needs, not temporary adjustments

- Building a functional relationship requires choosing sensory-friendly activities, timing events strategically, and accepting limitations

Chapter 7: Recognizing and Responding to Burnout

Supporting Recovery Without Enabling Avoidance

Your partner has been "off" for three weeks now. They're sleeping more than usual but still look exhausted. They've stopped doing hobbies they normally love. They're not returning texts from friends. Basic tasks—showering, cooking, leaving the house—seem to require enormous effort. You've asked what's wrong repeatedly. They say they don't know or they're just tired. You're frustrated because this looks like depression or laziness. You're tempted to push them to "snap out of it," get back to normal activities, force some routine. But something stops you. You sense this is different, though you can't quite explain how.

What you're witnessing might be autistic and ADHD burnout—a specific type of exhaustion that goes far deeper than regular tiredness or temporary stress. This isn't something your partner can just push through. And the strategies that work for typical stress or temporary fatigue can actually make burnout worse. Understanding the difference between burnout and other issues determines how you respond. Getting this wrong causes harm. Getting it right supports genuine recovery.

The Burnout Cycle in AuDHD

Burnout in AuDHD individuals follows a predictable pattern: accumulation, breakdown, recovery, and adaptation. This cycle often repeats throughout their lives, sometimes multiple times per year.

Accumulation phase: Your partner manages daily demands that exceed their actual capacity. They're masking at work, managing sensory input everywhere they go, forcing themselves through executive function tasks, pushing past social exhaustion. Each day they function "normally" costs more than they have to give. They're borrowing energy from tomorrow to get through today. This accumulation can last weeks, months, or even years. From the outside, they seem fine. Inside, they're running on empty and getting emptier.

Breakdown phase: The system crashes. Your partner can no longer maintain the facade of functioning. Skills they normally have suddenly disappear. They might lose the ability to speak in complete sentences, struggle with tasks they usually handle easily, or become unable to tolerate any sensory input. Their emotional regulation vanishes completely. Meltdowns and shutdowns happen frequently. They withdraw from everything and everyone. This isn't a choice or manipulation—it's neurological system failure under sustained overload.

Recovery phase: Your partner needs time and reduced demands to rebuild capacity. This phase requires rest, sensory calm, engagement with special interests, and minimal social demands. They're not being lazy. They're allowing their nervous system to recover from depletion. Forcing activity during this phase interrupts recovery and can extend burnout significantly.

Adaptation phase: Your partner gradually returns to functioning but often needs to make changes to prevent immediate re-entry into burnout. They might reduce work hours, establish firmer boundaries, or eliminate activities that contributed to the initial accumulation. These adaptations aren't temporary adjustments—they're permanent changes necessary to prevent cycling back into burnout.

This cycle is more severe in AuDHD individuals than in people with autism or ADHD alone. The combination creates faster accumulation, harder crashes, and longer recovery periods. Understanding this helps you recognize when your partner is in burnout versus experiencing other issues.

Recognizing True Burnout vs. Other Issues

Burnout has specific characteristics that distinguish it from depression, temporary stress, or laziness.

Chronic exhaustion that rest doesn't fix. Your partner sleeps eight hours and wakes up as exhausted as when they went to bed. Weekend rest doesn't restore them. Vacations don't help. The exhaustion is pervasive and unrelenting. This differs from regular tiredness, which improves with adequate rest.

Increased sensory sensitivity beyond their normal baseline. Sensory inputs that your partner usually tolerates become unbearable. Sounds hurt. Lights cause pain. Textures feel intolerable. Their sensory system has become hypersensitive because they lack the capacity to process even normal levels of input.

Severe executive dysfunction. Tasks your partner usually manages become impossible. They can't make decisions. They can't initiate activities. They can't follow multi-step processes. Their brain's management system has shut down to conserve energy.

Emotional dysregulation that's extreme even for them. Your partner cries over tiny things. They have meltdowns daily. They can't regulate emotional responses at all. Their emotional capacity has disappeared along with everything else.

Loss of masking ability. Your partner can no longer hide their autistic traits or ADHD symptoms. Stimming increases. Social skills vanish. They can't pretend to be neurotypical anymore because masking requires energy they don't have.

Complete social withdrawal. Your partner stops responding to messages, cancels all plans, and avoids even close friends and family. This isn't just needing alone time—it's inability to handle any social interaction.

Physical symptoms. Burnout often includes headaches, body aches, digestive problems, increased illness susceptibility, and other physical manifestations. The body is in distress, not just the brain.

Depression can coexist with burnout, but they're different. Depression involves persistent low mood, loss of interest in activities, feelings of worthlessness, and sometimes thoughts of self-harm. Burnout involves system-wide depletion and loss of capacity. Depression is about mood. Burnout is about capacity.

Laziness is about choosing not to do things you could do. Burnout is about being unable to do things you want to do. Your partner isn't choosing to avoid activities. They've lost the ability to engage in activities.

Case Example 1: The Three-Month Crash

Rebecca had been working full-time as a graphic designer for two years. She managed the sensory chaos of the open office, the social demands of meetings, the executive function challenges of project management. She came home exhausted every day but pushed through. She had a relationship, maintained friendships, kept her apartment clean. From the outside, she looked successful.

Her partner Zoe started noticing changes in October. Rebecca was more irritable. She stopped going to social events. She started ordering takeout instead of cooking. By November, Rebecca was coming home and immediately going to bed. She stopped responding to friends' texts. She cried frequently but couldn't explain why. By December, Rebecca called in sick to work multiple times. She couldn't get out of bed most days. She stopped showering regularly.

Zoe was confused and frustrated. Rebecca seemed depressed, but she insisted she wasn't sad—just utterly depleted. Zoe tried to help by suggesting activities, encouraging Rebecca to push through, and reminding her of responsibilities. This made things worse. Rebecca felt pressured and inadequate, which added stress without providing recovery.

What was happening: Rebecca was in full burnout. The accumulation phase had lasted two years. She'd been operating beyond her capacity that entire time, masking constantly, forcing herself through sensory and executive function challenges daily. Her system finally crashed. She entered the breakdown phase where basic functioning became impossible.

Zoe initially responded with strategies that work for temporary stress—stay active, maintain routine, push through. But burnout requires opposite responses. Rebecca needed permission to stop, rest, and recover without pressure. Once Zoe understood this was burnout, not depression or laziness, she could respond appropriately. She took over household tasks temporarily. She protected Rebecca from social demands. She allowed Rebecca to rest without guilt.

Recovery took four months. Rebecca gradually regained capacity. But she couldn't return to her previous life without changes. She negotiated remote work two days per week to reduce sensory demands. She established firmer boundaries with friends about last-minute plans. She built in more recovery time between activities. These adaptations prevented immediate return to burnout.

Case Example 2: The Cumulative Impact

David and his boyfriend Marcus had been together five years. Marcus had experienced several burnout episodes during that time, each lasting six to eight weeks. David noticed patterns: Marcus would push himself hard at work for months, saying yes to extra projects. He'd maintain a busy social calendar. He'd ignore signs of fatigue. Then he'd crash—suddenly unable to handle basic tasks, withdrawing completely, losing all capacity.

David felt increasingly frustrated with this pattern. Why wouldn't Marcus learn to pace himself? Why did he keep pushing until he broke? Why couldn't he prevent these crashes by managing his energy better? David started to feel like he was in a relationship with someone fundamentally unable to take care of themselves.

Here's what David didn't understand: Marcus's baseline capacity was lower than neurotypical people's, and his demands were higher. What looked like "normal life" to David actually exceeded Marcus's sustainable capacity. Marcus wasn't being reckless or irresponsible. He was trying to live a standard life with a non-standard nervous system. The crashes were inevitable given the mismatch between his capacity and his demands.

During one particularly severe burnout episode, Marcus and David had a serious conversation. Marcus explained that he genuinely couldn't perceive when he was approaching burnout until he was already in it. His autistic brain didn't send early warning signals David's neurotypical brain would send. His ADHD made it hard to remember to check in with himself about capacity. He wasn't ignoring signs—he literally didn't notice them.

They built a new system. David started tracking patterns Marcus couldn't see. "You've been working late every night this week and you had two social events last weekend. I'm noticing you're getting snappish and you're stimming more. What if we cleared this weekend for rest?" This external monitoring helped Marcus catch accumulation before breakdown.

They also accepted that burnout would still happen sometimes. Even with better monitoring, Marcus's life demands sometimes exceeded his capacity. Instead of fighting this reality, they planned for it. They built financial buffers for times when Marcus might need to reduce work hours. They established clear protocols for burnout episodes so David knew how to help without taking over completely.

Most importantly, David stopped viewing burnout as Marcus's personal failure. Burnout was a predictable response to operating beyond capacity in a world designed for neurotypical nervous systems. This reframe reduced David's frustration and Marcus's shame.

Case Example 3: The Postpartum Burnout

Aisha and her wife Kelly had a baby. The first few months were hard for everyone—sleep deprivation, constant demands, lifestyle upheaval. But while Kelly gradually adjusted, Aisha seemed to get worse instead of better. By month four, Aisha was barely functioning. She couldn't make decisions about what the baby should wear. She had meltdowns over which diaper to use. She stopped eating regularly. She couldn't tolerate the sound of the baby crying without noise-canceling headphones.

Kelly assumed this was postpartum depression. She urged Aisha to see a doctor. The doctor agreed it looked like postpartum depression and prescribed medication. But the medication didn't help. Aisha continued to deteriorate.

What was actually happening: Aisha was in severe burnout, not depression. The demands of new parenthood had overwhelmed her autistic and ADHD nervous system. The constant sensory input from baby sounds, the unpredictable schedule that destroyed routine, the executive function demands of managing baby needs, the loss of recovery time, the social isolation—all of this exceeded her capacity completely.

The baby's unpredictable crying triggered sensory overload multiple times per day. The disrupted sleep meant she never recovered from each day's demands. The executive function required to manage feeding schedules, diaper changes, doctor appointments, and household tasks while sleep-deprived became impossible. She was in constant accumulation with no recovery opportunity.

Kelly felt scared and alone. Aisha felt like she was failing at parenting. The medication didn't help because this wasn't primarily a mood disorder—it was capacity depletion.

Once they recognized this as burnout, they could respond appropriately. Kelly took over nighttime baby care completely so Aisha could sleep in a different room with earplugs and actually recover. They hired help for household tasks. They established a quiet space where Aisha could retreat when sensory overload hit. They accepted that Aisha's capacity for baby care was lower than expected and adjusted accordingly rather than forcing her to meet neurotypical parenting standards.

Recovery took six months. Aisha gradually rebuilt capacity, but she never reached the level of parenting involvement they'd initially imagined. She couldn't handle certain baby activities because they exceeded her sensory or executive function capacity. Instead of viewing this as failure, they divided parenting tasks based on what Aisha could actually handle. Kelly managed bath time and outings. Aisha handled quiet play and reading. They built sustainable parenting around Aisha's actual capacity rather than forcing her to meet idealized expectations.

Why Recovery Takes So Long

When people hear "burnout," they often think of typical workplace burnout that resolves with a week's vacation. AuDHD burnout is fundamentally different. Recovery doesn't happen in days or even weeks. It requires months or sometimes years.

Your partner's nervous system has been chronically depleted. They've been operating in survival mode for extended periods. Their brain has shut down non-essential functions to conserve energy. You can't rush neurological recovery any more than you can rush healing from major surgery. The system repairs at its own pace.

Forcing activity during recovery interrupts the healing process. Every demand on your partner requires energy they need for recovery. Social interaction, decision-making, sensory processing, emotional regulation—all of these consume the limited energy available. When you pressure your partner to "get back to normal," you're depleting resources needed for actual recovery.

Your partner might have good days during recovery where they seem almost back to normal. You might interpret this as recovery being complete. But burnout recovery isn't linear. Good days don't mean they're healed. Pushing them to maintain that good-day functioning often triggers setbacks that extend recovery.

The brain needs specific conditions to recover: reduced demands, minimal sensory input, engagement with interests that restore rather than deplete, social connection that doesn't require masking, and absence of pressure to perform. Creating these conditions for weeks or months is difficult when life doesn't stop for burnout. But attempting shortcuts extends the recovery timeline.

Common Causes You Can Address

Burnout develops from prolonged exposure to conditions that exceed capacity. Understanding these causes helps you identify changes that might prevent future burnout.

Masking exhaustion: Your partner suppresses natural autistic behaviors and mimics neurotypical presentation. This constant performance depletes them. Reducing environments where they must mask heavily provides relief. Home should be a place they can unmask completely.

Sensory overload: Chronic exposure to sensory input that overwhelms their system accumulates into burnout. Addressing sensory environment at home, choosing sensory-friendly activities, and building in sensory recovery time reduces this contributor.

Unmet needs: Your partner's needs for routine, special interests, quiet time, or specific accommodations go chronically unfulfilled. They keep functioning without getting what they actually need. Prioritizing their fundamental needs prevents accumulation.

Lack of understanding: When people around them don't understand or accommodate their neurodivergence, your partner expends extra energy explaining, justifying, or coping with invalidation. Your understanding and advocacy reduces this drain.

Excessive demands: Work expectations, social obligations, household responsibilities, and life admin overwhelm their executive function capacity. Reducing demands to match actual capacity prevents burnout accumulation. This might mean saying no to things other people handle easily.

You can't eliminate all these causes, but you can reduce their impact. Each reduction extends the time between burnout episodes and shortens recovery periods.

The Fundamental Needs Hierarchy

During burnout, your partner needs priorities clearly established. Not all needs are equal. Some are fundamental and must be met before others can be addressed.

Rest is non-negotiable. Sleep, stillness, reduced demands—these take priority over everything else. Your partner needs permission to rest without guilt or pressure. Rest isn't earned through productivity. It's required for recovery.

Sensory regulation comes next. Your partner needs calm sensory environments, ability to use sensory regulation tools, and freedom from sensory demands. This means accepting headphones indoors, dimmed lights, minimal sounds, and other accommodations without question.

Special interests provide restoration. Activities your partner hyperfocuses on aren't frivolous—they're recovery tools. Time spent on special interests restores capacity rather than depleting it. Allow and encourage this engagement even when it seems "unproductive."

Social support must be available without demands. Your partner needs to feel connected without having to perform socially. Your presence without expectation of conversation. Brief check-ins without lengthy discussions. Connection that doesn't require masking.

Other needs—household tasks, social obligations, work performance—come after these fundamental needs are addressed. Trying to maintain normal life while fundamental needs go unmet prolongs burnout indefinitely.

What Partners Can Do: Supporting Without Smothering

You want to help. But helping during burnout looks different than helping during temporary stress.

Be flexible with routines and plans. Routines that normally help your partner might feel impossible during burnout. Forcing adherence adds stress rather than providing comfort. Let them break routines without guilt. Plans you made can be canceled. Expectations can be adjusted. Flexibility demonstrates support.

Take over tasks temporarily—with clear communication. Your partner might need you to handle things they usually manage. This is different from the parent-child dynamic discussed earlier because it's time-limited and explicitly discussed. You both acknowledge this is temporary support during crisis, not permanent assumption of their responsibilities.

Protect them from external demands. Field phone calls, decline invitations on their behalf, run interference with family members who don't understand. Your partner lacks capacity to manage these things. You're not controlling them—you're creating the protected space they need for recovery.

Provide reassurance without pressure. Your partner probably feels guilty about being in burnout. They might worry you'll leave, think less of them, or get tired of supporting them. Regular reassurance that you're committed and this is temporary helps. But don't pressure them to "get better faster" while providing reassurance.

Learn their warning signs. Your partner might not notice they're approaching burnout. You can potentially catch accumulation earlier by tracking patterns they can't see. This isn't infantilizing—it's compensating for their difficulty with self-awareness around capacity.

Accept that recovery takes as long as it takes. Your frustration is understandable. But your partner can't speed up recovery to accommodate your timeline. Accepting this prevents additional pressure that interferes with healing.

What Partners Shouldn't Do: The Enabling Line

Supporting your partner during burnout doesn't mean eliminating all responsibilities forever or treating them as completely incapable.

Don't take over their entire life. They're in burnout, not helpless. They can still make decisions about what they need. They can still communicate boundaries. They can still contribute to the relationship in modified ways. Taking over everything reinforces helplessness and delays recovery.

Don't make burnout your responsibility to prevent. You can support and accommodate. You can help them recognize patterns. But ultimately, managing their capacity is their responsibility. You can't monitor their every activity and demand to prevent burnout. That's not sustainable for you.

Don't accept burnout as permanent. Sometimes partners in burnout resist recovery because burnout provides escape from demands. If your partner seems comfortable in burnout state and resistant to recovery, that's different from genuine healing. Recovery requires their active participation, not just passive rest indefinitely.

Don't eliminate all consequences. Your partner is still accountable for their behavior during burnout. They can't abuse you verbally and blame burnout. They can't completely neglect the relationship and expect you to accept it indefinitely. Burnout explains behaviors—it doesn't excuse all behaviors.

Don't abandon your own needs entirely. Supporting someone through burnout is draining. You need recovery too. You can't pour from an empty cup. Maintaining some attention to your needs isn't selfish—it's necessary for sustainability.

The line between supporting and enabling is: support removes barriers to recovery, enabling removes consequences of avoiding recovery.

Recognizing Your Own Burnout

While you're focused on your partner's burnout, you might develop your own. Partner burnout is a specific phenomenon affecting those who support neurodivergent individuals.

You feel chronically overwhelmed. Not just during crisis moments, but constantly. You're managing more than your share of relationship and household responsibilities. You're emotionally supporting your partner while receiving limited support yourself.

You're stressed and anxious frequently. You worry about triggering your partner. You monitor their mood and capacity constantly. You're hypervigilant about potential problems.

Physical symptoms develop: headaches, digestive issues, sleep problems, getting sick more often. Your body is responding to chronic stress.

You feel unappreciated. Your partner might not recognize how much you're doing because they're focused on survival. You feel taken for granted.

You're socially isolated. You've stopped seeing friends because you can't leave your partner or because explaining the situation is too exhausting.

You've lost yourself in the caretaking role. You can't remember the last time you did something just for yourself. Your identity has narrowed to "supportive partner."

If you're experiencing these symptoms, you're approaching or in burnout yourself. This requires action. You cannot support someone else from a depleted state. Your recovery is as important as theirs.

Preventing Both Partners' Burnout

Long-term relationship sustainability requires preventing burnout on both sides.

Build in regular recovery time for both partners. Your partner needs consistent downtime. You need consistent time away from caretaking. This isn't optional—it's structural requirement.

Distribute responsibilities based on actual capacity, not fairness. Your partner might contribute less to household management. This feels unfair until you recognize they're also managing invisible demands you don't have. Redefine fairness as "each person contributes what they can" rather than "each person contributes equally."

Maintain external support systems. You both need friends, hobbies, and interests outside the relationship. These prevent the relationship from becoming the only thing meeting all needs.

Communicate about capacity regularly. Don't wait until someone is in crisis. Check in about how much capacity each person has and adjust demands accordingly.

Accept professional help. Therapy, coaching, support groups— these aren't signs of failure. They're tools for sustainability. Use them before burnout, not just during crisis.

Prioritize the relationship alongside individual needs. Your partnership needs attention and care too. Build in time for connection that isn't about problem-solving or capacity management.

Moving Forward with Awareness

Burnout will probably happen again. Even with excellent management, your partner's capacity remains lower than neurotypical standards. Life will sometimes exceed that capacity. Instead of viewing this as failure, treat it as predictable event requiring prepared response.

You now understand what burnout looks like, what it needs, and how to support recovery without enabling avoidance. This knowledge helps you navigate future episodes with less confusion and more effectiveness. You can recognize accumulation earlier. You can respond appropriately during breakdown. You can support recovery without sacrificing your own wellbeing completely.

The next chapter addresses what happens when communication breaks down despite your best efforts—how to fight constructively when you inevitably hurt each other, misunderstand each other, or reach impasses that require resolution.

Understanding What You've Learned

- AuDHD burnout follows a predictable cycle of accumulation, breakdown, recovery, and adaptation that repeats throughout life

- Burnout involves chronic exhaustion, increased sensory sensitivity, severe executive dysfunction, emotional dysregulation, loss of masking ability, and social withdrawal

- Recovery requires months or years, not days or weeks, because the nervous system needs time to heal from chronic depletion

- Common causes include masking exhaustion, sensory overload, unmet fundamental needs, lack of understanding, and excessive demands

- During burnout, fundamental needs (rest, sensory regulation, special interests, social support) must be prioritized before other concerns

- Partners can support by being flexible with routines, temporarily taking over tasks, protecting from demands, and providing reassurance without pressure

- Partners should not take over completely, make burnout their responsibility to prevent, accept burnout as permanent, or eliminate all consequences

- Partner burnout is real and requires attention—you cannot support someone effectively from a depleted state

- Long-term sustainability requires regular recovery time, realistic responsibility distribution, external support systems, and capacity communication

- Burnout will likely recur, so preparation and planned responses are more realistic than attempting prevention

Chapter 8: Conflict Resolution Strategies

You asked your partner to please remember to lock the back door at night. It's the third time this week you've found it unlocked in the morning. You're trying to stay calm, but you're frustrated and concerned about safety. You say, "I really need you to lock the back door. This is important to me." Your partner immediately becomes defensive. "I'm trying! I forget sometimes! Stop acting like I'm doing it on purpose!" Their voice rises. You feel attacked when you were just expressing a reasonable need. You push back. "I'm not attacking you—I'm just asking you to lock the door!" They respond, "You're always criticizing me! Nothing I do is good enough!" Now you're both upset, voices raised, feelings hurt. A simple request about a door has become a relationship referendum. How did this happen?

Conflict in neurodiverse relationships escalates differently than in neurotypical relationships. The same neurological differences that create daily challenges also make resolving disagreements harder. Your different communication styles, emotional sensitivities, and perception filters turn minor issues into major fights. You both walk away feeling misunderstood and defensive. You both feel like you're the reasonable one and your partner is being difficult. And you're both probably right from your own perspective—which is exactly the problem.

Why Both Partners Feel Misunderstood

Research on neurodiverse relationships consistently finds that both partners feel chronically misunderstood. You feel like your partner doesn't get your perspective. They feel like you don't get theirs. This isn't one partner being difficult—it's genuine difference in how you each process the conflict.

You say something that seems perfectly clear and reasonable to you. Your partner hears criticism or rejection. They respond in a way that feels justified to them. You hear defensiveness or dismissal. You both escalate trying to be heard. Neither of you feels heard. Both of you feel attacked.

Here's what's happening neurologically: Your brains are literally processing the same interaction differently. The words you use carry different meanings in your respective brains. The tone you intend isn't the tone they perceive. The emotional context you're operating from isn't the context they're experiencing. You're having two different conversations using the same words.

Your neurotypical brain processes subtext, tone, and context automatically. When you say "I need you to lock the door," you mean exactly that—a specific request about a specific action. Your partner's neurodivergent brain might process this differently. The autistic part might hear criticism of their competence. The ADHD part might feel shame about their memory failures. The same sentence triggers completely different responses.

Your partner's direct communication style might feel harsh or critical to you when they mean it neutrally. They say "That doesn't work for me" and you hear rejection or dismissal. They meant a simple statement of fact. Your indirect communication might feel confusing or dishonest to them. You hint that you're upset, expecting them to notice. They take your words at face value and miss the subtext entirely.

Both of you are operating from your own neurological frameworks. Neither is more valid. But the mismatch creates constant miscommunication and escalation.

How to Communicate Concerns Without Triggering Defensiveness

The language you use during conflict matters enormously. Certain phrasings trigger defensive reactions before any productive discussion can happen.

Avoid "Why can't you ever..." or "How many times do I have to..." These phrases communicate frustration and criticism. They imply your partner is deliberately failing or incompetent. Even if you're legitimately frustrated, these phrasings shut down productive conversation immediately. Your partner hears "You're defective" rather than "This is a problem we need to solve."

Instead: "I need help solving this problem. The back door has been left unlocked several times. Can we figure out a solution together?"

Avoid "You always..." or "You never..." Absolute statements are rarely accurate and easy to defend against. Your partner can point to one exception and dismiss the concern entirely. Plus, these phrases feel like character attacks rather than behavior feedback.

Instead: "I've noticed a pattern that concerns me. The back door is often unlocked in the morning. I'm worried about security."

Avoid questions that are actually accusations. "Why didn't you lock the door?" sounds like a question but functions as criticism. You're not really asking for information—you're expressing displeasure. Your partner hears the criticism and responds defensively.

Instead: "I found the door unlocked again this morning. Can you tell me what makes this hard to remember?"

State your needs directly rather than complaining about their behavior. "I need to feel safe in our home, which means doors locked at night" is more productive than "You keep leaving the door unlocked." The first focuses on your need. The second focuses on their failure.

Use "I feel" statements carefully. These can be helpful but can also be manipulative if misused. "I feel unloved when you forget to lock the door" might be emotionally honest but puts huge weight on a practical issue. "I feel anxious about home security" communicates your emotional experience without making your partner responsible for fixing your feelings.

Acknowledge their effort even when addressing the problem. "I know you're trying to remember the door. I'm not questioning your effort. But this keeps happening and we need a different solution." This separates the problem from their worth as a person.

Case Example 1: The Dishes Debate Disaster

Leo was frustrated. His partner Mason left dirty dishes in the sink every day despite multiple conversations about it. Leo finally said, with clear frustration in his voice, "Why can't you just put your dishes in the dishwasher? It's not hard! I've asked you a million times!"

Mason immediately shut down. He went quiet, wouldn't make eye contact, and gave one-word responses. Leo felt ignored and dismissed. He pushed harder. "Are you even listening to me? This is exactly what I'm talking about! You don't care about what I need!" Mason exploded. "I'm done! Nothing I do is good enough for you! Maybe we shouldn't be together if I'm such a terrible partner!"

Leo was shocked. He'd just asked about dishes. How did this become relationship-ending? Mason stormed out and didn't come back for three hours. When he returned, he was calmer but couldn't explain why he'd reacted so intensely.

Here's what happened from Mason's perspective: He already felt shame about his executive function challenges. He genuinely tried to remember the dishes but failed regularly. When Leo said "Why can't you just..." Mason heard "This is easy and you're too incompetent to do it." When Leo added "I've asked a million times," Mason heard "You're a failure who can't do simple things."

The ADHD rejection sensitivity kicked in. Mason felt the criticism as devastating personal rejection. His autistic brain's black-and-white thinking went to "I'm a terrible partner and this relationship is doomed." His response wasn't proportional to dishes—it was proportional to the shame and rejection he experienced.

Leo had no idea his words triggered this cascade. He thought he was expressing reasonable frustration about a practical issue. But his language choice—"Why can't you just" and "It's not hard"—communicated judgment and criticism rather than collaborative problem-solving.

When they revisited this conversation later, they tried different language. Leo said, "The dishes are piling up and it's stressing me out. I know your brain doesn't remind you about this stuff. Can we figure out a system that works for both of us?" Mason could engage with this version because it didn't trigger rejection sensitivity. They installed a reminder on Mason's phone and agreed Leo would do a gentle check-in if dishes accumulated rather than letting frustration build.

The system wasn't perfect, but the conversation was productive rather than explosive.

Case Example 2: The Social Plans Spiral

Carmen made plans with friends for Saturday night. She mentioned it to her partner Jenna several times throughout the week. Saturday arrived. Carmen was getting ready. Jenna said, "I don't think I can go tonight. I'm too drained." Carmen felt hurt and annoyed. These were her close friends. Jenna had agreed to come. Now Carmen had to either cancel or go alone.

Carmen said, "You agreed to this. I've been talking about it all week. My friends are expecting both of us." Jenna responded, "I didn't realize how exhausted I'd be. I can't do it." Carmen pushed back. "You do this all the time! You agree to plans and then back out last minute. It's embarrassing!" Jenna got defensive. "I'm sorry I can't perform on command! If my limitations embarrass you, maybe you should find someone else!"

Both partners felt wronged. Carmen felt like Jenna didn't prioritize her needs or care about her friendships. Jenna felt like Carmen didn't understand or respect her capacity limitations. They went to the event together with tension between them the whole evening. Jenna spent the entire time miserable and overloaded. Carmen felt guilty for pressuring her but also resentful about the situation.

Here's what each partner experienced: Carmen wanted her partner involved in her social life. When Jenna agreed to plans, Carmen took that as commitment. Jenna's last-minute backing out felt like breaking a promise and not valuing Carmen's relationships. The pattern of agreeing then canceling made Carmen feel like she couldn't count on Jenna.

From Jenna's perspective: She agreed to plans with genuine intention to go. But her capacity fluctuated unpredictably. By Saturday, she'd spent all week managing sensory and social demands at work. She was approaching burnout. The thought of small talk and noise and social performance felt unbearable. She couldn't have predicted Monday how she'd feel Saturday. Her backing out wasn't breaking a promise—it was setting a necessary boundary based on actual capacity.

Both were right from their perspectives. Carmen had legitimate needs for reliability and social partnership. Jenna had legitimate capacity limitations that fluctuated. The conflict wasn't about who was wrong. It was about finding a way to honor both realities.

Their eventual solution: Jenna stopped committing to definite plans. Instead, she'd say "I'd like to try to make it but I can't promise until the day arrives." This felt uncomfortable to Carmen initially because she wanted commitment. But it was honest about Jenna's actual capacity. They also identified which events were truly important to Carmen. For those, Jenna would push herself more. For casual events, Carmen would make her own decision about attending without pressure on Jenna. This wasn't perfect for either partner, but it was functional.

Case Example 3: The Feedback Firestorm

Nate was working on a project at home. His partner Olivia walked past and commented, "Oh, you're using that approach? Interesting choice." She meant this neutrally—just observing. Nate immediately became defensive. "What's wrong with my approach? Do you think you could do it better? Why are you criticizing me?"

Olivia was surprised. "I wasn't criticizing! I was just making an observation!" Nate didn't believe her. "Your tone said it all. You think my approach is wrong." Olivia felt frustrated. "You're putting words in my mouth! I didn't say anything negative!" Nate shot back, "You didn't have to. I know when you're judging me."

They were both escalating. Olivia felt like she couldn't say anything without Nate taking it as an attack. Nate felt like Olivia criticized him constantly through supposedly "neutral" observations. Neither could understand the other's perspective.

Here's what was happening: Olivia's communication included subtext that she expected Nate to interpret. "Interesting choice" with a particular tone communicated her actual opinion. Neurotypical people would pick up this subtext automatically. Nate's autistic brain processed the literal words, not the tone. He heard "interesting choice" and interpreted that as neutral until he noticed Olivia seemed to expect a response beyond what the words warranted. This triggered suspicion that she meant something other than what she said, which felt dishonest and critical.

Nate's history of receiving criticism for his ADHD and autistic traits created hypersensitivity to any hint of judgment. Ambiguous communication triggered his rejection sensitivity because he interpreted ambiguity as hidden criticism.

They needed to change communication patterns from both sides. Olivia learned to state her actual thoughts directly rather than through implication. If she had concerns about Nate's approach, she'd say "I'm worried that approach might create problems because..." rather than "interesting choice." If she was truly neutral, she'd skip commentary that sounded like veiled judgment.

Nate worked on not assuming hidden criticism in neutral statements. But he also advocated for himself. "When you make observations about my work without clear feedback, I struggle to interpret your meaning. Can you tell me directly if you have concerns?" This gave Olivia specific information about what didn't work for him.

Focusing on Solutions Instead of Problems

Problem-focused language keeps you stuck in blame and defensiveness. Solution-focused language moves toward resolution.

Instead of: "Why are you always late?" **Try:** "Being on time is important to me. What would help you be ready earlier?"

Instead of: "You never help with housework!" **Try:** "I'm overwhelmed with housework. Can we divide tasks differently?"

Instead of: "You're on your phone constantly!" **Try:** "I need more present time together. Can we set phone-free hours?"

Notice the pattern. Solution-focused language:

- States your need clearly

- Invites collaboration

- Doesn't assign blame

- Focuses on future changes rather than past failures

This doesn't mean you can't express frustration. You can say "I'm really frustrated about this" before moving to solutions. But you follow frustration with "Let's figure out how to fix it" rather than dwelling on blame.

Your partner's neurodivergent brain often works better with concrete solutions than abstract feedback. "You need to be more considerate" is vague and feels judgmental. "Please text me if you're going to be more than 15 minutes late so I'm not worried" is specific and actionable.

The Power of Strategic Time-Outs

Conflicts escalate when emotional regulation fails. Once you're both flooded emotionally, productive conversation becomes impossible. Time-outs prevent escalation from reaching this point.

But time-outs only work if you've agreed on the system ahead of time. Spontaneous exits during arguments feel like abandonment or the silent treatment. Planned time-outs feel like self-care and relationship protection.

During a calm moment, discuss time-outs: "Sometimes we get too heated to communicate well. Can we agree that either of us can call a time-out if we're getting too emotional? We'll take 20 minutes apart, then come back and try again." Agree on how time-outs will be called. Maybe one partner says "I need a break" or you have a hand signal.

Establish rules: Time-outs are always honored without argument. The person who called it specifies when you'll reconvene. Both partners use the time to calm down, not to rehearse arguments. You return to the conversation unless you both agree to drop it.

Time-outs work because they interrupt escalation. Your partner's autistic brain might need time to process before they can respond thoughtfully. Your partner's ADHD brain might need time to calm emotional intensity before accessing rational thinking. Your neurotypical brain needs time to stop feeling defensive and return to empathy.

Twenty minutes can transform an explosive fight into a productive conversation. But only if both partners commit to the system before conflict arises.

Finding Humor in Miscommunications

Not all miscommunications need to become conflicts. Some can become inside jokes that strengthen your bond. This requires reframing miscommunications from "someone messed up" to "our brains are hilariously different."

Your partner takes an idiom literally and acts on it, creating absurdity. You asked them to "grab dinner" and they literally grabbed the dinner plates. Instead of frustration, you laugh together about the confusion. You build a collection of funny miscommunication stories.

You make plans using indirect communication. Your partner misunderstands completely. Instead of getting upset, you recognize the communication gap and find it amusing rather than annoying. "I said we should 'think about' going to that restaurant and you thought I meant today? Classic us!"

This reframe requires goodwill on both sides. You can't laugh at your partner's confusion in a way that feels mocking. They can't take offense at every miscommunication. But when you're both committed to finding humor in your differences, miscommunications become bonding opportunities rather than conflict triggers.

You develop catchphrases. "Lost in translation again!" becomes a gentle way to acknowledge miscommunication without assigning blame. You recognize patterns and joke about them. This doesn't fix the communication gaps, but it removes the emotional charge.

Avoiding Parent Trap Language During Fights

Chapter 4 discussed the parent-child dynamic that develops when you manage your partner's life. This dynamic also poisons conflict resolution. If you speak to your partner like a disappointed parent, they'll respond like a defensive child.

Parent trap language:

- "I shouldn't have to tell you this again."

- "How many times do we have to go through this?"

- "What were you thinking?"

- "I expected better from you."

- "This is unacceptable."

These phrases communicate judgment, superiority, and disappointment. They position you as authority and your partner as subordinate. Even if your frustration is legitimate, this language makes productive resolution impossible.

Partnership language:

- "This problem keeps coming up. Let's figure out why."

- "We've discussed this before and it's still happening. What's getting in the way?"

- "Help me understand what happened."

- "I'm disappointed about this. Can we talk about it?"

- "This isn't working for me. We need a different approach."

Partnership language treats your partner as an equal collaborator in solving shared problems. It doesn't minimize legitimate concerns, but it doesn't infantilize your partner either.

During conflict, monitor your tone and word choices. Are you speaking to an equal or lecturing a child? Are you collaborating or disciplining? Your partner will respond to the dynamic you create.

Understanding Different Perceptions of the Same Event

Here's something that helps: In neurodiverse conflicts, both partners can experience the same interaction completely differently and both be accurately reporting their experience.

You make a request. You experience it as reasonable and neutrally stated. Your partner experiences it as criticism and harshly delivered. You're both right about your own experience. Your brain processed the interaction as reasonable request. Their brain processed it as harsh criticism. The words were the same. The neurological processing was different.

Your partner asks for space. They experience this as a reasonable boundary. You experience this as rejection and withdrawal. You're both right about your experience. Their brain needed alone time for regulation. Your brain interpreted separation as relational threat.

This mutual validity of different experiences is hard to accept. You want to establish who was right. But there's no objective "right." There's your experience and their experience, both shaped by different neurological processing.

Accepting this changes conflict. Instead of "You misunderstood me" or "You're being too sensitive," you say "I experienced that one way and you experienced it differently. Let's figure out why and how to communicate better next time." Instead of establishing fault, you're identifying the gap between intention and impact.

Your intention doesn't override their impact. "I didn't mean it that way" doesn't erase their hurt. Their impact doesn't negate your intention. "You hurt me" doesn't mean you were trying to hurt them. Both are true simultaneously.

Repair Strategies After Conflicts

Healthy relationships aren't defined by avoiding conflict. They're defined by repairing effectively after conflict. Neurodiverse relationships need explicit repair strategies because indirect repairs often fail.

Apologize specifically. "I'm sorry I hurt you" is vague. "I'm sorry I said you never help with housework. That wasn't accurate and it dismissed your contributions" is specific. Your partner's autistic brain processes specific apologies better than general ones.

Acknowledge impact without defending intention. "I hear that my words hurt you. I didn't intend that, but I understand that's what happened" validates their experience while explaining yours. Don't use "but I didn't mean it" to erase their hurt.

Ask what they need. "What do you need from me right now to help repair this?" gives them agency. Some people need affection. Some need space. Some need discussion. Don't assume.

State what you'll do differently. "Next time I'm frustrated about housework, I'll ask if we can talk rather than expressing frustration directly" shows you're learning. Follow through on this commitment.

Check if repair is complete. "Are we okay?" or "Is there anything else we need to discuss about this?" confirms you've addressed the issue sufficiently. Don't assume silence means resolution for your autistic partner who might not signal needs clearly.

Don't drag up old conflicts during repair. "This is just like the time you..." prevents repair. Stay focused on the current issue. If patterns need discussion, address them separately during a calm time.

Accept that repair might take time. Your partner might need processing time before they're ready for repair. Forcing immediate resolution creates more problems. Give them space to regulate, then repair when both partners are ready.

Preparing for Future Conflicts

You can't prevent all conflicts. But you can set up systems that make conflicts less destructive.

Identify your personal triggers. When your partner knows you become defensive about X, they can approach X more carefully. When you know your partner becomes dysregulated about Y, you can discuss Y with extra sensitivity.

Establish ground rules. No name-calling. No bringing up past issues. No threats to end the relationship. Whatever boundaries make fights safer for both of you, establish them ahead of time and enforce them consistently.

Create a conflict check-in routine. Monthly or weekly, ask each other "How are we doing? Any concerns we should address?" This prevents small issues from becoming big fights because resentment accumulated.

Practice difficult conversations during calm times. Role-play how you'll discuss certain topics. This feels artificial but builds skills for actual conflicts.

Accept that some conflicts won't resolve. Some differences are fundamental. You need social stimulation; your partner needs social quiet. You value punctuality; their brain can't track time reliably. These gaps might not close completely. Success is managing them, not eliminating them.

Bridging to Partnership Wellness

You've learned to fight more fairly. But even healthy conflict is depleting. The next chapter addresses maintaining your own wellness while supporting your partner—how to prevent caretaker burnout, maintain your identity, and build support systems that sustain you through the challenges this relationship presents. Because you can't maintain a healthy partnership from a depleted self.

What You've Gained from This Chapter

- Both partners in neurodiverse relationships typically feel chronically misunderstood because different neurological processing creates genuinely different experiences of the same interaction

- Language choices dramatically impact conflict escalation; avoid "why can't you ever," "you always/never," and questions that are actually accusations

- Solution-focused language states needs clearly, invites collaboration, focuses on future changes, and avoids assigning blame

- Strategic time-outs prevent emotional flooding from making productive conversation impossible, but only if the system is agreed upon during calm times

- Finding humor in miscommunications reframes them as bonding opportunities rather than failures when both partners approach them with goodwill

- Parent trap language during fights positions one partner as authority and the other as subordinate, preventing equal partnership in problem-solving

- Both partners can accurately experience the same interaction completely differently; mutual validity of experiences is more productive than establishing who was "right"

- Effective repair requires specific apologies, acknowledging impact without defending intention, asking what they need, and committing to different future behavior

- Conflict preparation includes identifying triggers, establishing ground rules, creating check-in routines, and accepting that some fundamental differences won't resolve completely

Chapter 9: Building Your Support System

Maintaining Your Own Identity and Wellbeing

You're exhausted. You've been managing household tasks your partner can't handle. You're monitoring their mood and capacity constantly. You're fielding questions from family members who don't understand why your partner "can't just" do normal things. You're explaining, advocating, protecting, accommodating. Meanwhile, your own needs have been on the back burner for so long you can barely remember what they are. You haven't seen friends in weeks. You've stopped doing hobbies you used to love. You're snapping at people at work. You're not sleeping well. You feel resentful but guilty about the resentment. And you're wondering how long you can keep this up.

This is partner burnout. It's real, it's common, and it can destroy relationships even when both partners love each other. You can't sustain a healthy partnership from a depleted self. You can't support someone else indefinitely while neglecting your own wellness. The airline safety announcement gets it right: put on your own oxygen mask before helping others. But somehow in relationships, especially when your partner has obvious struggles, this wisdom feels selfish. It's not. It's survival.

The Statistics on Partner Distress

Research on relationships affected by ADHD and autism consistently shows that non-neurodivergent partners experience significantly higher levels of frustration, stress, and relationship distress compared to partners in neurotypical relationships.

Studies find that partners of individuals with ADHD report nearly twice as much relationship dissatisfaction. Partners of autistic individuals describe feeling lonely, socially excluded, and chronically misunderstood.

You're not imagining the extra difficulty. The challenges you face are objectively harder than what most couples manage. You're dealing with executive function deficits that create more household burden. You're managing emotional dysregulation that requires constant emotional labor. You're accommodating sensory needs that limit your activities. You're explaining neurological differences to everyone who questions why things work differently in your relationship.

The relationship failure rate for partnerships involving ADHD is nearly twice as high as relationships without ADHD. This isn't because love isn't present or commitment isn't real. It's because the practical and emotional demands exceed what many partners can sustain long-term without proper support and self-care.

Understanding these statistics isn't depressing—it's validating. Your struggles aren't personal failure. They're predictable response to objectively challenging circumstances. And recognizing the challenge is the first step toward building sustainable strategies.

Recognizing Your Own Burnout

Partner burnout looks different from but shares characteristics with the burnout your neurodivergent partner experiences. Learn to recognize your own symptoms.

You feel overwhelmed most of the time. Not just during crisis moments. Constantly. You wake up tired and go to bed exhausted. The to-do list never ends. You feel like you're drowning in responsibilities.

Stress and anxiety are your baseline. You're always slightly worried about the next problem, the next meltdown, the next thing your partner will forget. You can't fully relax because you're mentally preparing for what might go wrong.

Physical symptoms appear. Headaches, digestive problems, muscle tension, frequent illnesses, sleep disruption. Your body is responding to chronic stress that your mind might be minimizing.

You feel unappreciated and taken for granted. Your partner might not notice how much you're doing because they're focused on their own struggles. You feel invisible and undervalued.

Resentment builds despite love. You love your partner and don't want to feel resentful. But you're angry about carrying disproportionate responsibility. The resentment creates guilt, which creates more stress.

Social isolation increases. You've stopped seeing friends. Partly because you're too tired. Partly because explaining your relationship situation is exhausting. Partly because you can't leave your partner alone too long. Your social world has shrunk dramatically.

You've lost your identity beyond this relationship. When someone asks about you, your mind goes blank. Who are you besides your partner's support system? You can't remember. Your hobbies, interests, and goals have disappeared under the weight of caretaking.

You fantasize about escape. Not necessarily leaving the relationship. But imagining a week alone. A day where nothing needs managing. Time where you're not responsible for anyone's wellbeing. These fantasies feel shameful but they're signals of deep depletion.

If multiple symptoms resonate, you're in or approaching burnout. This requires immediate action, not eventually-when-things-calm-down action. Things won't calm down on their own. You have to create calm.

Case Example 1: The Disappearing Self

Alicia and her partner Jonas had been together for seven years. Jonas had ADHD and autism. Alicia had gradually absorbed more and more household management. She scheduled everything, managed finances, handled all social communication, organized their lives. She also worked full-time, maintained relationships with both their families, and tried to provide emotional support when Jonas had meltdowns or periods of low mood.

Alicia's friend Rachel noticed Alicia never seemed available anymore. When they did manage to meet, Alicia spent the entire time talking about Jonas's latest struggle or complaining about forgotten tasks. Rachel gently pointed out that Alicia seemed to have disappeared. "Who are you besides Jonas's partner? What do you want? What do you care about?" Alicia couldn't answer.

She'd stopped painting, which she'd loved. She'd quit the book club. She'd stopped running. She couldn't name a hobby or interest that was hers alone. Her identity had narrowed to "person who manages Jonas's life and compensates for his challenges." She'd lost herself completely in the caretaking role.

Rachel's questions triggered something. Alicia realized she was miserable, resentful, and depleted. She loved Jonas but hated her life. She needed to rebuild herself alongside the relationship.

Alicia started small. She committed to painting one hour per week, non-negotiable. Jonas could manage the house for one hour. She joined a painting class, which also provided social connection outside the relationship. She started running again, which provided stress relief and time alone. She established a weekly coffee date with Rachel where they discussed Alicia's life, not just Jonas's challenges.

Jonas initially resisted these changes. He felt abandoned when Alicia wasn't available. He struggled with the additional responsibility of managing things during her painting time. But Alicia held firm. "I need this to stay healthy. A healthy me makes our relationship work better." She was right. As Alicia rebuilt her identity and interests, her resentment decreased. She had more emotional capacity for Jonas because she was getting her own needs met.

Case Example 2: The Isolation Trap

Marcus was married to Simone, who had significant sensory sensitivities and social difficulties. Social events drained Simone quickly, so Marcus and Simone rarely attended gatherings together. Marcus started declining invitations because explaining why Simone couldn't come was exhausting. His friends stopped inviting him. His social circle shrank.

Marcus worked from home, so he didn't have workplace social connections. Simone was essentially his only social contact. He felt isolated and lonely but couldn't articulate this to Simone because he didn't want to make her feel bad about her limitations.

The isolation affected Marcus's mental health. He felt depressed and trapped. He started resenting Simone even though the situation wasn't her fault. Their relationship suffered because Marcus couldn't be emotionally present when he was depleted and isolated.

Marcus finally talked to Simone. "I'm lonely. I need social connection outside our relationship. This isn't about you being inadequate—it's about me needing more people in my life." Simone was hurt initially but recognized Marcus's need was legitimate.

They built a new system. Marcus accepted invitations to social events alone. Simone encouraged this rather than feeling threatened by it. Marcus joined a weekly basketball game with friends. He started meeting a friend for breakfast once a month. These connections restored Marcus's emotional wellbeing and actually improved the relationship. He wasn't placing all his social and emotional needs on Simone anymore.

Case Example 3: The Anxiety Spiral

Tasha's partner Dev had ADHD. Dev forgot appointments, left tasks unfinished, and struggled with time management. Tasha found herself constantly anxious, mentally tracking Dev's obligations and reminding them about commitments. She checked whether Dev had completed tasks. She worried about what Dev might forget next. She felt responsible for preventing Dev's failures.

This anxiety consumed Tasha's mental energy. She couldn't focus at work because she was worrying about whether Dev remembered their doctor appointment. She couldn't relax in the evening because she was mentally reviewing tomorrow's schedule to catch potential forgotten items. She was exhausted from the constant mental load.

Tasha's anxiety also created tension. Dev felt micromanaged and criticized. Tasha felt like she couldn't stop monitoring because Dev would forget important things. They were locked in an unhealthy dynamic where Tasha's anxiety drove controlling behaviors that made Dev feel inadequate, which reinforced Tasha's belief that she had to manage everything.

Tasha talked to a therapist about this pattern. The therapist helped her recognize she was carrying responsibility that wasn't hers. Dev was an adult. Dev's forgetting had consequences, but those were Dev's consequences to manage, not Tasha's to prevent.

Tasha worked on letting go. She stopped reminding Dev about most things. She stopped checking whether tasks were complete. She allowed Dev to experience natural consequences of forgotten commitments. This felt terrifying initially. Wouldn't everything fall apart?

Some things did fall apart. Dev missed appointments. Dev forgot to pay a bill. But Dev also learned. The natural consequences motivated Dev to build better systems. Dev started using phone reminders more consistently. Dev asked Tasha for help with specific things rather than Tasha assuming responsibility for everything.

Tasha's anxiety decreased significantly. She wasn't carrying mental load that wasn't hers anymore. The relationship improved because they'd shifted from anxious-parent and irresponsible-child to two adults managing their own lives.

The Critical Importance of Self-Care

Self-care isn't selfish. It's not indulgent. It's not optional. It's the foundation that makes everything else possible.

You cannot support someone else from an empty tank. You cannot be emotionally present in your relationship when you're depleted. You cannot make good decisions when you're exhausted and resentful. You cannot maintain patience and compassion when your own needs are chronically unmet.

Self-care creates a healthier you, which creates a more resilient relationship. When you're rested, you respond to your partner's challenges with understanding rather than frustration. When your emotional needs are being met through multiple sources, you're not dependent on your partner for all emotional support. When you have outlets for stress, you don't explode at your partner over small issues.

Your partner also benefits from your self-care. They don't want to destroy you. They don't want you depleted and resentful. Most neurodivergent partners recognize their needs create extra demands on you. Your self-care removes the guilt they might feel about burdening you. It proves the relationship is sustainable.

Self-care isn't bubble baths and face masks (though those are fine too). Self-care is:

- Saying no to things that deplete you
- Maintaining friendships and social connections
- Pursuing hobbies and interests outside the relationship
- Getting adequate sleep and exercise
- Seeking therapy or support when needed
- Setting and enforcing boundaries
- Taking time alone without guilt

Self-care requires deliberate, protected time. It doesn't happen in leftover moments. You schedule it the same way you schedule anything important.

Maintaining Individual Identity

You are not just your partner's support system. You're a complete person with your own interests, goals, values, and needs. Maintaining this identity is essential.

Pursue hobbies independently. You need activities that are yours alone. Activities that engage you, challenge you, or bring you joy without involving your partner. This might be art, sports, reading, gaming, music, volunteering, or anything else that lights you up. Protect time for these activities as non-negotiable.

Maintain friendships outside the relationship. You need people who know you beyond your role as someone's partner. People who are interested in your thoughts, feelings, and experiences separate from relationship dynamics. These friendships provide perspective, support, and connection that can't come from your partner.

Set personal goals unrelated to the relationship. What do you want to achieve professionally? Physically? Creatively? Intellectually? These goals give you direction and motivation beyond keeping the relationship functional.

Spend time alone. Not just away from your partner—truly alone. Time with your own thoughts without managing anyone else's needs. This might be walks, meditation, solo activities, or just sitting quietly. Alone time helps you stay connected to yourself.

Maintain your values and interests. Don't abandon things that matter to you because they're not compatible with your partner's needs. Find ways to honor your values even if you have to do it differently than you imagined. You value community involvement but your partner can't handle crowds? Volunteer in ways that don't require them. You love travel but your partner struggles with unfamiliar environments? Take some trips solo or with friends.

Losing yourself in a relationship creates resentment and dependency. Maintaining yourself creates sustainability and authenticity.

Finding Alternative Support Systems

Your partner cannot be your only source of emotional support, practical help, and social connection. You need multiple sources.

Friends provide social connection and perspective. Talk to friends about your life—not just your relationship challenges, but your experiences, thoughts, and feelings about everything. Friends remind you that you're more than your partner's support system. They provide validation, advice, and companionship.

Family might offer practical support. Depending on your family dynamics, relatives might help with tasks, provide respite, or offer financial assistance during difficult times. Family connection also maintains your identity beyond this single relationship.

Support groups connect you with others facing similar challenges. Online or in-person support groups for partners of neurodivergent individuals provide understanding that friends and family might not offer. These people get it. They validate your struggles without judgment. They offer practical strategies based on lived experience. You don't have to explain or justify.

Therapy provides professional support. Individual therapy gives you space to process your experiences, develop coping strategies, and maintain mental health. A therapist helps you recognize unhealthy patterns, set boundaries, and care for yourself without guilt. Therapy isn't admission of failure—it's commitment to wellness.

Community involvement provides purpose and connection. Volunteering, joining clubs, participating in religious communities, or engaging with interest groups gives you identity and belonging outside the relationship. You contribute to something meaningful beyond managing household dynamics.

Professional help for practical tasks reduces your burden. Housekeepers, accountants, meal delivery services, virtual assistants—outsourcing tasks that drain you creates space for activities that restore you. Money spent on these services is investment in relationship sustainability.

You might feel guilty about needing other people. You might think a good partner should be enough. But humans need community. Neurodiverse relationships require especially strong support networks because the challenges are objectively greater. Building this network isn't betraying your partner—it's building foundation that sustains the relationship long-term.

Setting Clear Boundaries

Boundaries protect your wellbeing without abandoning your partner. They define what you can sustainably give and what exceeds your capacity.

Time boundaries: "I need two evenings per week for my own activities." "I'm not available for late-night conversations about this issue—we'll discuss it tomorrow." "I need one weekend per month to myself."

Emotional boundaries: "I'll listen and support you, but I can't fix this for you." "I can't process your emotions while also managing my own—I need a break." "Your meltdowns aren't acceptable reasons to treat me poorly."

Task boundaries: "I'll help with X, but Y is your responsibility." "I can't take on more household management—we need to outsource or lower standards." "I won't call to remind you about appointments anymore."

Communication boundaries: "I need us to have this conversation when I'm not already stressed." "I can't discuss this topic right now—let's schedule time later." "I need written communication about complex topics because verbal overwhelms me."

Setting boundaries feels uncomfortable initially, especially if you've been accommodating endlessly. Your partner might react negatively. They might feel abandoned or accused. Hold firm. Boundaries aren't punishment—they're requirements for your sustainable participation in the relationship.

Explain boundaries clearly: "I need time for myself not because I don't love you, but because I'll resent you if I don't get it. These boundaries protect our relationship." Most neurodivergent partners can understand this logic even if they initially feel hurt.

Enforce boundaries consistently. If you set a boundary and don't maintain it, your partner learns the boundary is negotiable. Consistency proves you're serious.

When to Seek Professional Help

Couples therapy provides structured support for relationship challenges. Individual therapy addresses your personal wellbeing. Both are valuable.

Seek couples therapy when:

- Communication has broken down completely
- Conflicts escalate regularly despite your best efforts
- Resentment is damaging your connection
- You're considering ending the relationship
- You need help navigating a major transition
- You want to build better patterns proactively

Find a therapist experienced with neurodiverse relationships. General couples therapy doesn't always address the specific challenges you face. A therapist who understands autism and ADHD can provide targeted strategies rather than generic relationship advice.

Seek individual therapy when:

- You're experiencing depression, anxiety, or other mental health symptoms
- You're struggling to cope with relationship demands

- You need support developing boundaries

- You're losing your sense of self

- You need space to process without involving your partner

- You want to work on your own patterns that contribute to problems

Therapy isn't failure. It's investment in wellness. Many people wait until crisis before seeking help. Proactive therapy prevents crisis and builds skills during calmer times.

You're a Team: Mutual Responsibility

You support your partner with their neurological challenges. But they also have responsibility to manage their condition and support you.

Your partner should be:

- Actively working on strategies to manage executive function, emotional regulation, and other challenges

- Seeking treatment appropriate for their needs (therapy, coaching, medication if relevant)

- Communicating clearly about their needs and limitations

- Recognizing and appreciating your efforts

- Making efforts to meet your needs even when difficult for them

- Taking responsibility for their behaviors rather than blaming neurodivergence for everything

You're not responsible for managing your partner's condition. You support them, but they must do the work of understanding themselves, building coping strategies, and actively participating in making the relationship functional.

If your partner isn't doing their part—if they're passive about their challenges, unwilling to develop strategies, or expecting you to manage everything—the relationship is unsustainable. You can't make someone participate in their own wellness. Partnership requires both people contributing their best efforts.

Have explicit conversations about mutual responsibility. "I'm committed to understanding and accommodating your needs. I need you committed to managing your symptoms and meeting my needs too. We're both responsible for making this work." This conversation might feel confrontational, but it's necessary.

Looking Toward Thriving

You've spent chapters learning about challenges: executive function deficits, emotional dysregulation, sensory sensitivities, burnout, conflict patterns. You've built understanding of what makes these relationships difficult. The final chapter shifts focus. How do you build a relationship that doesn't just survive but actually thrives? How do you celebrate the unique strengths of your partnership? How do you create long-term sustainability and genuine happiness together?

Core Principles to Carry Forward

- Non-neurodivergent partners experience objectively higher stress and relationship dissatisfaction in neurodiverse relationships, validating that your struggles are real and predictable

- Partner burnout symptoms include chronic overwhelm, anxiety, physical symptoms, resentment, social isolation, lost identity, and escape fantasies requiring immediate attention

- Self-care isn't selfish—it creates a healthier you, which creates a more resilient relationship with greater capacity for challenges

- Maintaining individual identity through independent hobbies, friendships, personal goals, alone time, and preserved values prevents resentment and codependency

- Alternative support systems (friends, family, support groups, therapy, community involvement, professional services) provide necessary emotional and practical resources beyond what your partner can offer

- Clear boundaries around time, emotions, tasks, and communication protect your wellbeing without abandoning your partner when communicated clearly and enforced consistently

- Couples therapy for relationship challenges and individual therapy for personal wellbeing are investments in sustainability, not admissions of failure

- Your partner has equal responsibility to manage their condition, develop strategies, appreciate your efforts, and work toward meeting your needs

Chapter 10: Thriving Together

Celebrating Strengths and Building a Neurodiverse Partnership That Works

You've read nine chapters about challenges. Executive function deficits that create household chaos. Emotional dysregulation that feels like walking on eggshells. Sensory sensitivities that limit your activities. Burnout cycles that deplete you both. Communication gaps that turn minor issues into major fights. Partner exhaustion that threatens the relationship foundation. It's been heavy. Real. Necessary. But here's what you also need to know: neurodiverse relationships aren't just problem collections requiring constant management. They have unique strengths. They offer gifts that neurotypical relationships don't provide. And they can be deeply satisfying, authentic partnerships where both people thrive.

This isn't Pollyanna optimism. This is recognition that the same neurological differences creating challenges also create strengths. The same traits that frustrate you also bring value. Your relationship isn't broken. It's different. And different offers possibilities that "normal" doesn't.

The Unique Strengths You Have Access To

Neurodiverse relationships provide experiences and benefits that many neurotypical partnerships lack. These aren't consolation prizes for dealing with difficulties. These are genuine advantages.

No masking required between partners. Your AuDHD partner can be completely themselves with you—no suppressing stims, no forcing eye contact, no pretending to care about small talk, no monitoring every behavior. The relief of this authenticity is profound. They can finally rest at home instead of performing constantly. This creates deeper intimacy than many neurotypical relationships achieve because your partner isn't hiding fundamental parts of themselves.

Mutual understanding of being different. Both partners understand what it's like to not fit standard expectations. You might be neurotypical, but you've chosen a non-standard relationship. You've learned to think outside conventional boxes. You both understand that "normal" isn't the only way or the best way. This shared understanding of being outside mainstream creates strong connection.

Complementary skills and perspectives. Your partner's autistic attention to detail catches things you miss. Their ADHD creativity generates solutions you wouldn't think of. Their different way of processing information provides alternative perspectives on problems. Your neurotypical social skills handle situations they struggle with. Your executive function manages areas where they get stuck. You're not just managing deficits— you're combining genuinely different strengths.

Authentic connection without pretense. Many relationships operate on unspoken rules, implications, and social performance. Your relationship can't function that way because your partner processes communication differently. This forces more genuine interaction. You say what you mean. You address issues directly. You can't hide behind politeness or implication. This directness creates deeper authenticity.

Building your own relationship rules. You can't follow standard relationship scripts because those don't work for your partner's brain. This freedom allows you to design relationship structures that actually serve you both rather than conforming to what relationships "should" look like. You have permission to be creative because conventional wasn't an option anyway.

Shared weird acceptance. Your partner's special interests might seem odd to others. Your partner's needs might seem excessive to others. But in your relationship, weird is normal. This creates safety to be fully yourselves without judgment. You both get to be accepted for who you actually are, not who you're supposed to be.

These strengths are real. Notice them. Name them. Celebrate them. They're not small things—they're the foundation of partnership that many people spend their lives seeking but never find.

How Differences Create Balance

The same differences that create friction also create balance when you stop fighting against them.

Routine provides stability; novelty provides stimulation. Your partner's autistic need for routine prevents life from becoming chaotically reactive. Your partner's ADHD need for novelty prevents life from becoming boring stagnation. Together you maintain structure that's flexible enough to stay interesting.

One partner's weakness is the other partner's strength. You struggle with big-picture thinking. Your partner sees patterns and connections easily. Your partner struggles with detailed planning. You handle logistics well. Instead of both people having identical capabilities, you cover each other's gaps.

Different energy patterns complement each other. Your partner might be useless in the morning but energized at night. You might be morning-productive but exhausted by evening. Instead of both partners needing the same schedule, you can divide responsibilities based on natural energy patterns.

Emotional intensity balances emotional steadiness. Your partner feels things deeply and passionately. You remain calm during emotional storms. This combination handles both the highs of passionate engagement and the stability of steady presence. Neither alone provides complete range—together you access full emotional spectrum.

Different social needs prevent codependency. Your partner needs significant alone time. You need social connection. Instead of both partners requiring identical levels of togetherness, you each get what you need without the other feeling neglected or smothered. This built-in independence actually strengthens the relationship.

Divergent thinking plus linear thinking equals better problem-solving. Your partner's neurodivergent brain approaches problems from unexpected angles. Your brain follows logical sequences. Combining these approaches solves problems neither of you would solve alone.

These aren't accommodations or compromises. These are genuinely complementary patterns that create more functional partnership than two neurotypical people with identical processing might create.

Real Couples: How They've Learned to Complement

Reading about strengths in abstract helps. Seeing how actual couples leverage their differences helps more.

Dividing labor based on actual brains: One couple divided household responsibilities completely contrary to gender expectations. The autistic partner handled all planning, scheduling, and detailed organization because their brain excelled at systems. The neurotypical partner handled all social communication, last-minute adjustments, and relationship maintenance because their brain managed social dynamics easily. Neither partner did work their brain struggled with. Both contributed meaningfully from their strengths.

Using hyperfocus productively: One couple recognized the ADHD partner's hyperfocus capability as superpower rather than problem. Major household projects—renovations, deep cleaning, complex research—got assigned to the ADHD partner during hyperfocus periods. The neurotypical partner handled steady maintenance that required consistency. This division meant both types of work got done by the person whose brain fit the task.

Communication repair through scripts: One couple created scripts for common conflicts. When the autistic partner felt overwhelmed, they used predetermined phrase: "System overload—need reboot." The neurotypical partner knew this meant give space, reduce demands, check back later. No explanation required. No hurt feelings about withdrawal. The script allowed communication during times when communication capacity was gone.

Celebrating special interests together: One couple turned the autistic partner's intense special interests into shared activities. The neurotypical partner learned about the topics and engaged genuinely, not just tolerating. This created deep bonding over subjects most people found boring. The special interests became relationship glue rather than solitary escape.

Parallel play as quality time: One couple redefined togetherness. They'd sit in the same room, each doing separate activities, occasionally sharing thoughts. This counted as quality time because they were sharing space and choosing to be together even while independently engaged. No forced interaction. No entertainment of each other. Just comfortable coexistence.

Energy management through explicit communication: One couple tracked each person's daily capacity. Morning check-in:

"How's your tank today?" High capacity days meant taking on extra household or emotional work. Low capacity days meant the other partner covered more. This flexible distribution based on actual current capacity prevented resentment about "equal" splits that ignored reality.

Appreciation for different processing: One couple learned to value different problem-solving approaches. Neurotypical partner approached problems systematically and socially. Neurodivergent partner approached problems creatively and independently. When facing decisions, they'd explicitly use both approaches and combine insights. Different became advantage rather than obstacle.

Maintaining Emotional and Physical Intimacy

Intimacy requires effort in any long-term relationship. In neurodiverse relationships, intimacy requires intentional adaptation to different needs.

Sharing experiences in compatible ways: Traditional date nights might not work if your partner finds restaurants overwhelming. But hiking, visiting quiet museums, working on projects together, or engaging with special interests side-by-side creates shared experience without sensory overload. Intimacy comes from time together, not from specific activities.

Spending quality time on each other's terms: Sometimes quality time looks like what your partner needs—sitting quietly in the same room with minimal interaction. Sometimes it looks like what you need—active conversation and focused attention. Taking turns honoring each other's version of connection maintains balance.

Expressing appreciation regularly and specifically: "Thank you for being you" might feel good but means little to an autistic brain that processes concrete information better than abstract sentiment. "Thank you for doing the dishes even though I know executive function makes starting tasks hard. That helped me feel supported today" provides specific, meaningful appreciation.

Physical touch that works for both: Your partner might not like light touch but crave deep pressure. They might love specific kinds of physical connection but find others intolerable. Instead of assuming touch preferences, explicitly discover and honor what actually feels good to their nervous system. Physical intimacy that causes sensory distress isn't intimacy.

Emotional intimacy through honesty: Many relationships maintain emotional distance through politeness and implication. You can't do that because your partner's brain doesn't process implication. This forces more honest emotional communication, which creates deeper intimacy once you adjust to the directness.

Accepting that intimacy fluctuates: Your partner's capacity for connection varies with burnout, stress, and sensory state. Instead of demanding consistent levels of intimacy, accept the natural ebb and flow. High-intimacy periods are intense and connecting. Low-intimacy periods provide recovery. Both are necessary phases of sustainable partnership.

Dividing Tasks by Strengths, Not Equality

Functional neurodiverse relationships abandon "fair" in favor of "functional." Fifty-fifty splits don't work when partners have dramatically different capacities in different areas.

Assign tasks based on who can actually do them well: Your partner with strong autistic systematizing handles finances, schedules, detailed planning. You handle social coordination, last-minute flexibility, emotional support to family members. Neither person does work their brain struggles with unless absolutely necessary.

Accept unequal contribution without resentment: You might handle 70% of household tasks because your partner's executive function can't maintain consistent task completion. This feels unfair until you recognize your partner is also managing 100% of dealing with discrimination, masking demands, sensory assault, and executive function challenges you don't experience. "Equal" is impossible to measure across such different experiences.

Value invisible labor: Your partner's autistic organizational skills might create household systems that save everyone time. Your neurotypical social skills might maintain family relationships that your partner couldn't manage. These contributions aren't visible the way washing dishes is visible, but they're equally valuable.

Trade off rather than split: One partner manages area A entirely while the other manages area B entirely. Clean division prevents both partners trying to collaborate on tasks where collaboration creates communication overhead that exceeds individual effort.

Outsource the areas neither partner handles well: Some tasks don't fit either brain. Instead of fighting over who has to do the thing neither person can do successfully, outsource it. Hire services, use technology, lower standards, or eliminate the task. Not everything must be done by partnership labor.

Recognize different contribution styles: Your partner might contribute in intense bursts during hyperfocus but contribute nothing during other periods. You might contribute steadily. These different patterns provide equal value over time even though they look different week to week.

Creating Relationship Structures That Work for You

Standard relationship expectations don't apply. You get to build partnership rules that fit your actual needs.

Define your own version of quality time: Society says quality time means focused interaction, conversation, eye contact. Your partnership might define quality time as being in the same room while independently engaged, taking walks in comfortable silence, or parallel activities that don't require conversation. Your definition is valid if it works for both of you.

Establish communication systems that fit your brains: Many couples resolve conflicts through discussion. You might need written communication for complex topics. You might need predetermined scripts for common issues. You might need processing time between discussion rounds. Build systems around how your brains actually communicate, not how brains "should" communicate.

Design social life that accommodates both partners: You might attend some events together and others separately. You might host small gatherings instead of attending large ones. You might have shorter social engagement limits than other couples. Your social patterns should work for your actual partnership, not match what you see other couples doing.

Accept non-traditional relationship timelines: Your partner might need slower relationship escalation because change is difficult. You might live separately longer than typical. You might not follow standard life milestones on expected schedule. Your timeline is yours to set.

Create space for independence within connection: Many relationships emphasize togetherness as primary value. Your relationship might emphasize individual autonomy with chosen connection. Your partner needs significant alone time. You need independent activities. Instead of viewing this as lack of closeness, view it as sustainable interdependence.

Lower standards where needed: Not everything must be done to conventional standards. Your house might be messier than others because energy gets allocated to more important things. Your social etiquette might be nonstandard. Your schedules might be unconventional. If it works for you both, it's fine.

Building Trust, Vulnerability, and Safety

Deep partnership requires feeling safe with each other. In neurodiverse relationships, safety requires specific attention because misunderstandings threaten it constantly.

Consistent communication about needs: Both partners stating clearly what they need, when they need it, without expecting mind-reading. This consistency builds trust that needs will be met because they're clearly expressed.

Following through on commitments: When executive function is challenged, follow-through is harder. But reliability builds trust. When your partner says they'll do something and they do it, trust grows. When you say you'll accommodate something and you do, trust grows. Building systems to support follow-through protects trust.

Vulnerability about struggles: Your partner being honest about when they're overwhelmed, approaching burnout, or struggling with symptoms. You being honest about when you're frustrated, depleted, or need more support. This vulnerability prevents resentment from building silently.

Accepting each other's limitations without judgment: Your partner can't do everything they wish they could. You can't meet every need your partner has. Accepting these limitations without making them character flaws creates safety. "This is hard for my brain" gets met with "I know, let's figure out accommodations" rather than "you should try harder."

Repairing ruptures explicitly: Every couple has conflicts and hurts. Repairing explicitly rather than assuming time heals everything maintains trust. Direct apology, clear commitment to change, follow-up to ensure repair was sufficient—these protect connection.

Celebrating victories together: When your partner manages something their brain struggles with, celebrate it. When you successfully navigate a challenging situation, acknowledge it together. Shared celebration of progress builds positive association and hope.

Long-Term Strategies for Sustainable Partnership

Building a relationship that lasts requires looking beyond immediate problems to structural sustainability.

Regular relationship check-ins: Monthly or quarterly, assess how things are working. What's going well? What needs adjustment? What upcoming challenges need preparation? These check-ins catch small issues before they become relationship threats.

Continuing education about neurodivergence: Both partners keep learning about autism, ADHD, and how they manifest in relationships. Understanding evolves. New strategies emerge. Staying current maintains effectiveness.

Maintaining individual growth alongside relationship growth: Both partners need personal development separate from relationship development. You're both growing as individuals, which allows growth as partners. Stagnant individuals create stagnant relationships.

Building financial sustainability: Neurodiverse partnerships might need accommodations that cost money—therapy, services, reduced work hours, outsourced tasks. Financial planning that accounts for these needs prevents crisis and enables necessary supports.

Creating community support: Relationships exist in context. Building community that understands and supports your partnership—friends who get it, family who've learned, support groups, therapists—provides safety net for difficult times.

Planning for transitions: Life changes—job shifts, moves, health issues, potential children. Transitions are especially hard for autistic individuals. Planning ahead, discussing concerns, building support for transitions maintains stability.

Accepting that hard times will come: Some periods will be harder than others. Burnout will recur. Conflicts will happen. Life will present challenges. Accepting this as normal rather than sign of failure helps you weather difficult periods without panic.

The Power of Curiosity Over Control

One mindset shift transforms neurodiverse relationships: approaching differences with curiosity rather than attempting to control or fix them.

Control says: "Why can't you just be on time?" Curiosity says: "What makes timekeeping difficult for your brain? How can we work around that?"

Control says: "You need to get over your sensory issues." Curiosity says: "What does sensory overload feel like for you? What helps?"

Control says: "Your way is wrong." Curiosity says: "Your way is different. Help me understand it."

Control creates resistance and resentment. Curiosity creates understanding and collaboration. Control assumes there's a right way (usually the neurotypical way). Curiosity recognizes multiple valid approaches.

When your partner does something that seems illogical or frustrating, curiosity asks: "What's the logic in your brain that made that choice make sense?" Often there is logic—just different logic based on different neurological processing. Understanding that logic helps you work with it rather than against it.

Curiosity also applies to self: "Why does this particular behavior trigger me so strongly? What need am I trying to meet? What assumption am I making?" Your reactions aren't always about your partner's behavior—sometimes they're about your expectations, past experiences, or unmet needs that you're projecting onto the situation.

Compassion Over Criticism

Related to curiosity: approaching challenges with compassion rather than criticism transforms relationship quality.

Your partner forgot something important. Criticism says: "How could you forget? This is unacceptable!" Compassion says: "I can see you're frustrated with yourself. Let's figure out how to prevent this next time."

Your partner has a meltdown over something that seems small. Criticism says: "You're overreacting." Compassion says: "You're overwhelmed right now. What do you need?"

Your partner can't do something most people find easy. Criticism says: "Everyone else manages this." Compassion says: "This particular thing is especially hard for your brain. How else might we approach it?"

Criticism creates shame spirals that make functioning harder. Compassion creates safety that allows vulnerability and growth. Your partner already lives with daily evidence that their brain works differently and struggles with things others find easy. Your criticism adds nothing constructive. Your compassion provides environment where they can acknowledge challenges and work on them.

Compassion doesn't mean avoiding accountability. Your partner is still responsible for their behavior. But you can hold people accountable compassionately: "I understand why this happened, and it's still not okay. We need to figure out how to prevent it because it affects me negatively." Compassion and boundaries coexist.

Resources for Continued Learning

This book has provided foundation. But learning shouldn't stop here. Neurodiverse relationships require ongoing education as you discover new challenges and strategies.

Books on neurodiverse relationships: Multiple books address autism-neurotypical partnerships, ADHD relationship challenges, and specific aspects of neurodivergent love. Reading diverse perspectives provides different strategies and validation.

Online communities: Forums, social media groups, and discussion boards connect you with others navigating similar challenges. These communities offer real-time support, practical advice, and reminder that you're not alone.

Therapy and coaching: Professionals specializing in neurodiverse relationships can provide personalized guidance. Couples therapy, individual therapy, and relationship coaching all offer value. Don't wait for crisis—proactive support prevents problems.

Educational resources about autism and ADHD: Understanding the neurological foundations of your partner's experiences helps you interpret behaviors correctly. Blogs, podcasts, videos, and articles by neurodivergent people themselves provide insider perspective.

Workshops and conferences: Events focused on neurodiversity, autism, or ADHD provide concentrated learning and community connection. Both in-person and virtual options exist.

Your partner's direct teaching: Your partner is the expert on their experience. Ask them about their internal process. Let them teach you about how their brain works. This direct communication often provides more useful information than any book.

Your Path Forward

You started this book confused, frustrated, probably exhausted. You've learned about executive function challenges, emotional dysregulation, sensory processing differences, burnout cycles, communication gaps, and partner wellness. You've gained tools for navigating these challenges more effectively.

But more than tools, you've gained perspective. Your partner's behaviors aren't character flaws or deliberate difficulties. They're neurological realities. Your relationship challenges aren't signs of incompatibility or failure. They're predictable results of different brain wiring operating in a world designed for one type of brain.

You can't eliminate the challenges. AuDHD doesn't disappear. But you can build relationship structures that work with these realities rather than against them. You can develop communication systems that bridge different processing styles. You can divide labor based on actual capabilities. You can recognize burnout early and respond effectively. You can maintain your own wellness alongside supporting your partner.

Most importantly, you can recognize that your relationship isn't just problem management. It offers unique strengths, authentic connection, and partnership possibilities that many people never experience. The challenges are real. But so are the rewards.

You're not just surviving this relationship. You're building something genuine, creative, and potentially extraordinary. You're proving that love doesn't require identical brains. You're demonstrating that different can be better than normal.

Keep learning. Keep adapting. Keep celebrating what works. Keep caring for yourself. Keep appreciating your partner's unique brain. Keep building partnership that honors you both.

You've got this. And you're not doing it alone.

What This Final Chapter Has Shown You

- Neurodiverse relationships offer unique strengths including authentic connection without masking, complementary skills, freedom to create original relationship structures, and shared acceptance of being outside mainstream norms

- Neurological differences that create friction also create balance when you stop fighting against them—routine and novelty, different strengths covering weaknesses, varied energy patterns, emotional range, and problem-solving from multiple approaches

- Successful neurodiverse couples divide labor based on actual brain capabilities, use predetermined communication systems, turn special interests into bonding opportunities, redefine quality time, and manage energy explicitly

- Maintaining intimacy requires sharing experiences in compatible ways, expressing appreciation specifically, physical touch that works for both partners' nervous systems, honest emotional communication, and accepting fluctuation in connection capacity

- Functional task division abandons fifty-fifty equality in favor of assigning responsibilities based on who can actually do them well, accepting unequal visible contribution, valuing invisible labor, and outsourcing what neither partner handles effectively

- Creating relationship structures that work for you means defining your own versions of quality time, communication systems, social life, relationship timelines, independence within connection, and standards that serve your partnership

- Building trust and safety requires consistent communication about needs, following through on commitments, vulnerability about struggles, accepting limitations without judgment, repairing ruptures explicitly, and celebrating victories

- Long-term sustainability strategies include regular relationship check-ins, continuing education about neurodivergence, maintaining individual growth, building financial sustainability, creating community support, planning for transitions, and accepting that difficult periods will occur

- Approaching differences with curiosity instead of control and compassion instead of criticism transforms relationship quality by creating understanding and collaboration rather than resistance and resentment

- Ongoing learning through books, online communities, therapy, educational resources, workshops, and direct communication with your partner provides continued support and strategy development

Appendix A: Red Flags vs. AuDHD Traits

Red Flags (Potential Abuse/Unhealthy Dynamics):

- Deliberately manipulating you using their diagnosis as excuse

- Refusing to take any responsibility for managing symptoms

- Using meltdowns to control your behavior or punish you

- Isolating you from friends and family

- Consistently dismissing your needs while demanding accommodation of theirs

- Showing no interest in how their behaviors affect you

- Using diagnosis to justify cruel or disrespectful treatment

- Refusing therapy or support while expecting you to manage everything

AuDHD Traits (Neurological Differences):

- Forgetting tasks and appointments despite trying to remember

- Sensory sensitivities that limit activities

- Need for significant alone time to recharge

- Difficulty reading social cues and nonverbal communication

- Emotional dysregulation during overwhelm

- Executive function challenges with planning and organization

- Taking language literally and missing implied meanings

- Inconsistent social energy and engagement

Key Difference: Traits are neurological patterns that cause struggle for both partners. Red flags are choices that benefit one partner at the other's expense. Traits improve with understanding and accommodation. Red flags worsen without accountability.

Appendix B: Communication Scripts for Difficult Conversations

Expressing a Need: "I need [specific thing]. This matters to me because [reason]. Can we talk about how to make this happen?"

Addressing a Recurring Problem: "[Specific issue] keeps happening. I know you're not doing it on purpose. Can we figure out why it's hard to change and build a system that works better?"

Setting a Boundary: "I need [specific boundary] to stay healthy in this relationship. This isn't negotiable, but I'm open to discussing how we implement it in a way that works for both of us."

Requesting Time to Cool Down: "I'm getting too emotional to have a productive conversation. I need [specific amount of time] to calm down. Can we come back to this at [specific time]?"

Initiating Repair After Conflict: "I'm sorry I [specific behavior]. That wasn't okay. I understand it affected you by [specific impact]. Next time I'll [specific change]. Is there anything else you need from me to repair this?"

Discussing Capacity: "My tank is at [percentage] today. That means I can handle [what you can do] but not [what you can't do]. What's your capacity today?"

Addressing Burnout Concerns: "I'm noticing [specific signs] which makes me think you might be approaching burnout. Can we talk about what's contributing and what might help?"

Appendix C: Crisis Plan Template for Meltdowns/Shutdowns

Prevention:

- Early warning signs to watch for: _____
- Triggers to avoid when possible: _____
- Preventive strategies that help: _____

During Meltdown:

- DO: _____
- DON'T: _____
- What helps most: _____
- How long to give space before checking in: _____

During Shutdown:

- DO: _____
- DON'T: _____
- Communication alternatives (gestures, written): _____
- How long shutdowns typically last: _____

Recovery:

- What helps recharge after episode: _____

- When to discuss what happened: _____

- How to know when recovery is complete: _____

Emergency Contacts:

- Therapist: _____

- Trusted friend/family: _____

- Crisis line if needed: _____

Appendix D: Self-Care Checklist for Partners

Daily:

- [ ] Get adequate sleep (7-9 hours)

- [ ] Eat regular, nourishing meals

- [ ] Take at least 15 minutes completely alone

- [ ] Do one small thing just for yourself

- [ ] Move your body in some way

Weekly:

- [ ] Spend time with friend(s) outside the relationship

- [ ] Engage in hobby or interest independently

- [ ] Have at least one conversation not about partner/relationship

- [ ] Assess your own energy and capacity levels

- [ ] Do something that restores you

Monthly:

- [ ] Evaluate relationship patterns and address concerns

- [ ] Check whether boundaries are being maintained

- [ ] Assess whether support systems are adequate

- [ ] Review whether you're losing yourself in caretaking

- [ ] Plan something to look forward to

Signs You Need More Self-Care:

- Feeling resentful frequently
- Physical symptoms (headaches, digestive issues, tension)
- Can't remember last time you did something for yourself
- Feeling anxious or overwhelmed constantly
- Social isolation increasing
- Lost connection to your own interests and goals

Appendix E: Resource Directory

Books:

- *ADHD & Us* by Anita Robertson
- *The Couple's Guide to Thriving with ADHD* by Melissa Orlov
- *Autism and Relationships* resources from various authors
- *Is This Autism?* by Donna Henderson, Sarah Wayland, and Jamell White
- *Neurodiversity at Work* by Amanda Kirby and Theo Smith

Websites:

- CHADD (Children and Adults with Attention-Deficit/Hyperactivity Disorder): chadd.org
- Embrace Autism: embrace-autism.com
- Neurodivergent Insights: neurodivergentinsights.com
- ASAN (Autistic Self Advocacy Network): autisticadvocacy.org

- ADDA (Attention Deficit Disorder Association): add.org

Online Communities:

- Reddit: r/AspiePartners, r/ADHD_partners
- Facebook groups for neurodiverse relationships
- Online forums specific to autism and ADHD relationships

Finding Therapists:

- Psychology Today therapist directory (filter for ADHD/autism specialties)
- AANE (Asperger/Autism Network) provider directory
- Local autism organizations often have provider lists
- Ask for recommendations in online support groups

Support Groups:

- Local CHADD support groups for partners
- Autism society local chapters often have partner support
- Online support groups through various organizations
- Consider starting your own if none exist locally

References

- 3SC. (2025). When ADHD meets neurotypical: The challenges in relationships (and how to overcome them). 3SC.

- Acevedo, B. P., Aron, E. N., Aron, A., Sangster, M.-D., Collins, N., & Brown, L. L. (2014). The highly sensitive brain: An fMRI study of sensory processing sensitivity and response to others' emotions. *Brain and Behavior, 4*(4), 580–594.

- ADDA. (2024). ADHD spouse burnout: Essential strategies for lasting support. ADD Association.

- ADDitude Magazine. (2025). Autism and relationships: Neurodiverse couples' strengths, complements. ADDitude.

- American Psychiatric Association. (2013). *Diagnostic and statistical manual of mental disorders* (5th ed.). American Psychiatric Publishing.

- Aron, E. N., & Aron, A. (1997). Sensory-processing sensitivity and its relation to introversion and emotionality. *Journal of Personality and Social Psychology, 73*(2), 345–368.

- Aron, E. N., Aron, A., & Jagiellowicz, J. (2012). Sensory processing sensitivity: A review in the light of the evolution of biological responsivity. *Personality and Social Psychology Review, 16*(3), 262–282.

- Autism.org.uk. (n.d.). Autism and communication. National Autistic Society.

- Backer van Ommeren, T., Koot, H. M., Scheeren, A. M., & Begeer, S. (2015). Reliability and validity of the Interactive Drawing Test: A measure of reciprocity for children and adolescents with autism spectrum disorder. *Journal of Autism and Developmental Disorders, 45,* 2007–2018.

- Barkley, R. A. (1997). Behavioral inhibition, sustained attention, and executive functions: Constructing a unifying theory of ADHD. *Psychological Bulletin, 121*(1), 65–94.

- Barkley, R. A. (1997). *ADHD and the nature of self-control.* Guilford Press.

- Bottema-Beutel, K., Yoder, P., Warner, C., & Crowley, S. (2014). The role of supported joint engagement and parent utterances in language and social communication development in children with autism spectrum disorder. *Journal of Autism and Developmental Disorders, 44,* 2162–2174.

- Boterberg, S., & Warreyn, P. (2016). Making sense of it all: The impact of sensory processing sensitivity on daily functioning of children. *Personality and Individual Differences, 92,* 80–86.

- CHADD. (2021). Don't give up, don't give in: Survival skills for the non-ADHD partner. *Attention Magazine.* Children and Adults with ADHD.

- Cortese, S., Adamo, N., Del Giovane, C., Mohr-Jensen, C., Hayes, A. J., Carucci, S., ... Cipriani, A. (2018). Comparative efficacy and tolerability of medications for attention-deficit hyperactivity disorder in children, adolescents, and adults: A systematic review and network meta-analysis. *The Lancet Psychiatry, 5*(9), 727–738.

- Embrace Autism. (2023). Coping with AuDHD burnout. Embrace Autism.

- Embrace Autism. (2023). Preventing AuDHD burnout. Embrace Autism.

- Engel-Yeger, B., & Ziv-On, D. (2011). The relationship between sensory processing difficulties and leisure activity preference of children with different types of ADHD. *Research in Developmental Disabilities, 32*(3), 1154–1162.

- Faraone, S. V., & Biederman, J. (2005). What is the prevalence of adult ADHD? Results of a population screen of 966 adults. *Journal of Attention Disorders, 9*(2), 384–391.

- Faraone, S. V., Sergeant, J., Gillberg, C., & Biederman, J. (2003). The worldwide prevalence of ADHD: Is it an American condition? *World Psychiatry, 2*(2), 104–113.

- Freelife Behavioral Health. (2025). From spark to shutdown: AuDHD burnout. Freelife Behavioral Health.

- Gottman Institute. (2024). Two different brains in love: Conflict resolution in neurodiverse relationships. The Gottman Institute.

- Healthline. (2025). Have a partner with ADHD? 10 tips for offering support. Healthline.

- HelpGuide.org. (2024). Adult autism and relationships. HelpGuide.

- HelpGuide.org. (2025). Adult ADHD and relationships. HelpGuide.

- Higgins, J. M., Arnold, S. R. C., Weise, J., & Pellicano, E. (2020). Defining autistic burnout through experts by lived experience: Grounded Delphi method investigating #AutisticBurnout. *Autism, 25*(8), 2356–2369. *(Use the journal's final publication year if your database lists a different year.)*

- Huang, Z., Wang, P., et al. (2024). Relationships between sensory processing and executive functions in children with combined ASD and ADHD compared to typically developing and single-disorder groups. *Frontiers in Psychology, 15*, Article ID (e-pub).

- Jagiellowicz, J., Aron, A., & Aron, E. N. (2016). The trait of sensory processing sensitivity and neural responses to changes in visual scenes. *Social Cognitive and Affective Neuroscience, 11*(7), 1031–1038.

- Julien Nathanson Counselling. (2025). Burnout and shutdown: The hidden cost of living as an AuDHD person. Julien Nathanson Counselling.

- Kern, J. K., Trivedi, M. H., Garver, C. R., et al. (2007). Sensory correlations in autism. *Autism, 11*(2), 123–134.

- LA Concierge Psychologist. (2025). Five ways to avoid autism-related communication problems in adult relationships. LA Concierge Psychologist.

- Lai, S.-S., et al. (2020). Identifying the cognitive correlates of reciprocity in children with autism spectrum disorder. *Journal of Autism and Developmental Disorders, 50*, 2007–2018.

- Lau, W. Y., & Peterson, C. C. (2011). Adults and children with Asperger syndrome: Exploring adult attachment style, marital satisfaction and satisfaction with parenthood. *Research in Autism Spectrum Disorders,* *5*(1), 392–399.

- Love on the Autism Spectrum. (2025). Emotional intimacy for neurodiverse couples. Love on the Autism Spectrum.

- Love on the Autism Spectrum. (2025). Effective communication in neurodiverse relationships. Love on the Autism Spectrum.

- Mansour, R., Dovi, A. T., Lane, D. M., Loveland, K. A., & Pearson, D. A. (2017). ADHD severity as it relates to comorbid psychiatric symptomatology in children with autism spectrum disorders (ASD). *Research in Developmental Disabilities, 60*, 52–64.

- Milestones Autism Resources. (n.d.). Interacting with autistic people. Milestones.

- Milton, D. E. M. (2012). On the ontological status of autism: The "double empathy problem." *Disability & Society, 27*(6), 883–887.

- Neurodivergent Insights. (n.d.). ADHD burnout recovery: What helps and what makes it worse. Neurodivergent Insights.

- Neurodivergent Insights. (n.d.). Autism and ADHD burnout: Signs, symptoms, and support. Neurodivergent Insights.

- Neurodiverse Couples Counseling. (n.d.). Autism meets ADHD: Can polar opposites make great partners? Neurodiverse Couples Counseling.

- Orlov, M. (2025). Marriage communication tips for spouses of ADHD adults. *ADDitude Magazine*.

- Panagiotidi, M., Overton, P., & Stafford, T. (2020). The relationship between sensory processing sensitivity and ADHD traits: A spectrum approach. *ADHD Attention Deficit and Hyperactivity Disorders, 12*(1), 89–98.

- Psychology Today. (2020). Making sense of sensory overload in autism and ADHD. Psychology Today.

- Psychology Today. (2024). Time blindness. Psychology Today.

- Relational Psych Group. (2025). How autistic people experience romantic relationships differently. Relational Psych Group.

- Robertson, A. E., & Simmons, D. R. (2013). The relationship between sensory sensitivity and autistic traits in the general population. *Journal of Autism and Developmental Disorders, 43*(4), 775–784.

- Raymaker, D. M., Teo, A. R., et al. (2020). "Having all of your internal resources exhausted beyond measure and being left with no clean-up crew": Defining autistic burnout. *Autism in Adulthood, 2*(2), 132–143.

- Sagebrush Counseling. (2025). Autistic and ADHD as a couple. Sagebrush Counseling.

- Shimmer ADHD Coaching. (2024). My partner doesn't understand ADHD. Shimmer.

- STAR Institute. (n.d.). Sexuality through the senses: 15 ways disordered sensory processing affects intimacy. STAR Institute for Sensory Processing.

- Talkspace. (2025). ADHD spouse burnout: How to cope. Talkspace.

- The Autism Service. (2025). ADHD and relationships. The Autism Service.

- UCI Health. (2024). Coping with time blindness and ADHD. UCI Health.

www.ingramcontent.com/pod-product-compliance
Lightning Source LLC
Chambersburg PA
CBHW071224290326
41931CB00037B/1958